THE
LEARNING
OF
MOTOR SKILLS

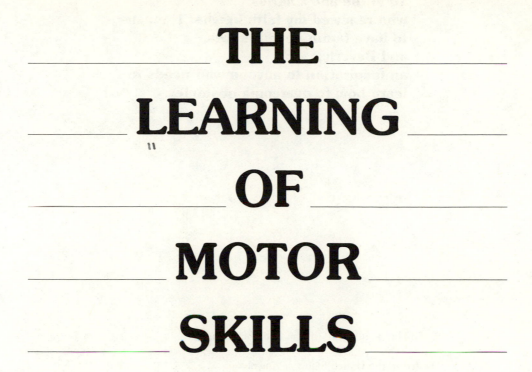

THE
LEARNING
OF
MOTOR
SKILLS

ROBERT N. SINGER

The Florida State University

Macmillan Publishing Co., Inc.
New York

Collier Macmillan Publishers
London

To Millie and Charles,
who renewed my faith in what it means
to have family togetherness,
and Beverly,
an inspiration to anyone who needs to
learn how to overcome obstacles.

Macmillan Publishing Co., Inc.
866 Third Avenue, New York, New York 10022

Collier Macmillan Canada, Ltd.

Library of Congress Cataloging in Publication Data
Singer, Robert H.
  The learning of motor skills.
  Includes bibliographical references and index.
  1. Physical education and training. 2. Motor
ability—Study and teaching. 3. Learning,
Psychology of. I. Title.
GV341.S494   613.7'1   81–8154
ISBN 0–02–410790–5   AACR2

Printing: 1 2 3 4 5 6 7 8   Year: 2 3 4 5 6 7 8 9 0

PREFACE

The learning of movement skills, such as sports activities, is of interest to all of us, as participants, teachers, or both. The challenge is to understand learning processes and conditions in order to teach and learn as productively as possible. But how? Where do we begin?

Learning and teaching effectiveness depend on many considerations. In this book we attempt to formulate guidelines that should be helpful in many ways. Although dependent upon research and theory, the intent is to be as practical as possible. Documentation is at a minimum. With the use of many examples, especially from sports, descriptions of learning processes and prescriptions for instructional procedures serve as the basis of the contents in this book.

The psychology of learning is rich with implications and indications as to those factors that contribute best to achievement. Not only are there guidelines for people in general but for individual difference considerations as well. Any study of learning must account for similarities and meaningful differences among people.

In addition, we can analyze learning at the most sophisticated level or at a more applied level. Since this may be your first experience with material dealing with learning, and your orientation will probably be to use it to be a more capable teacher or coach, there is little reason in this book for us to be too concerned with jargon, semantics, and theory. Abstract material can be simplified and practical relevance determined. It is hoped that this book will be useful as a solid introduction to learning, to benefit your teaching and learning experiences.

Learning and teaching are more fun when desirable outcomes are realized quickly and painlessly. We are no longer at a point where we should be satisfied to proceed by trial and error. Indeed, learning can proceed in a reasonably orderly and predictable manner, when proper considerations are made in practice. Practice in itself does not make perfect. It should be good practice. When ideal situational conditions are present, and learners are motivated appropriately, the results are much more favorable.

For many years, physical educators and coaches have realized that there is a strong relationship among the behavioral sciences, the applied sciences, and physical education and sport. Such recognition is leading to more applications of scientific information in curricula, instruction, and training.

This book may serve several purposes. Primarily it is designed as a textbook for a motor learning course. However, it may well be utilized as a reference source for a methods course, a foundations course, a principles course, coaching courses, and your own needs in teaching and learning various skills.

In the preparation of the book, an over-riding guideline was to present the material in a manner that should make it easy to digest. Documentation and technical terminology have been kept to a minimum. There are more discussions of and references to specific research toward the middle and end of the book. This plan is meant to lead the reader gently into the world of behavioral research, without a feeling of being overwhelmed. It should be emphasized, however, that there exists a substantial body of knowledge associated with many of the topics covered in this book. The more interested student will read other sources to broaden the depth of understanding of a particular topic.

The book serves as a foundation for a more advanced book in motor learning, entitled *Motor Learning and Human Performance: An Application To Motor Skills and Movement Behaviors* by the same author, now in its third edition (1980), published by the Macmillan Publishing Co.

R.N.S.

CONTENTS

1

PERSPECTIVES ON LEARNING   1

2

DIRECTIONS IN RESEARCH AND THEORY   19

3

THE MEASUREMENT OF LEARNING 35

4

MOTOR LEARNING ACTIVITIES AND TASKS 55

5

THE ACQUISITION OF SKILL 81

6

ESTABLISHING PRACTICE CONDITIONS 103

9

THE HIGHLY SKILLED   185

10

MOTOR LEARNING AND PROGRAMS OF PHYSICAL EDUCATION AND SPORT   209

11

AN OVERVIEW: LEARNING PRINCIPLES   217

1

PERSISTENCE

PERSPECTIVES

ON

LEARNING

It's incredible! Think about it. Think about what we have learned and accomplished. Think about what we will probably be learning in the near future and the distant future. We, as human beings, have tremendous capabilities to learn and to master many kinds of activities.

Oh, yes, there are frustrations. There have been occasions when we have not come to close to attaining the level of achievement that we would have liked. If we think back to very early years, there were times when we probably felt that we never would be able to hit a ball, throw it, or kick it in any effective manner. But we did. Later we would tackle more complex sports. These involved some of the simpler skills, but now they were sequenced and organized in a more complicated manner. Again, we probably felt we would never learn them. But we did. Sure, some people learned faster and better than others in some activities. Some had more fun than others in the process of learning. Whether we realized it or not, we learned not only skills and information, but also about the learning process: how it works for us as individuals and how we each could benefit from certain conditions.

Learning doesn't have to be haphazard or occur by chance. Furthermore, it can be enjoyable. As a prospective teacher or coach, your primary mission will be to help others learn and attain a sense of fulfillment. You will be responsible for their learnings, feelings, and overall development. That's quite a challenge. But it is a challenge that can be met.

1

TEACHING AND LEARNING

What Is Taught?

It is obvious that physical education teachers and coaches teach athletic and recreational skills. They teach, and students learn, to perform movements and to perfect skills. If rules and strategies are involved, these must be taught as well.

But we often take for granted the learning of appropriate attitudes, motivations, and feelings that will contribute to skilled performance. These must be taught and learned, too. Thus, performance level in movement skills is a result of learning that has taken place for that movement, but also of the condition of the body, the control and direction of emotions and motivation, and the ability to cope with whatever problems arise. When we recognize that the learning of skills involves so many considerations, we can better understand how complex teaching and learning can be. Obviously, however, better educated and more sensitive teachers and coaches should be able to produce more favorable outcomes for the students in their programs than should those who are less capable and motivated.

How To Teach?

It would be nice if there were one blueprint for teaching. But this is not the case. There are many acceptable approaches, and preference depends on each teacher's personal philosophy, personal teaching style, objectives, situations, and the like. But underlying *any* approach should be *scientific principles of learning*. Teaching need not, and indeed should not, proceed in an unorganized way. It should be well planned and thought out. It should reflect what is known about learners in general, perceived differences among individual learners, and improved learning conditions for all the students.

What Is Learned?

Learning happens all the time. Indeed, it can occur right after birth. Much of our learning, both intentional and accidental, comes about through observation and imitation of others. Classes and athletic programs are usually associated with more formal ventures into learning. Consequently, we should expect the best conditions for learning to be present in formal programs; that is, objectives should be obtained more efficiently and effectively under the guidance of professionals.

In such formal programs, learning will reflect the emphasis placed by the teacher on the attainment of certain objectives, be they primarily physical development, the learning of skills, the learning of social behaviors, or the development of self. Therefore, it is important for the teacher to consider objectives, instructional emphasis, and the nature of the students in the particular setting when instruction is planned.

TYPES OF LEARNING

Many kinds of learning can be influenced in situations. We as physical educators are typically concerned with *movement learning*, more formally termed *motor learning* and *psychomotor behaviors*. And yet, it is often apparent that students need to learn rules and regulations, tactics, equipment maintenance, and possibly the history of the sport. These would typically be considered as *cognitive behaviors*. Furthermore, we try to develop appropriate attitudes in students toward activity, as well as techniques to deal with emotions so that they work for the person instead of against the person in learning and performing skills. Emotions and attitudes typically are referred to as *affective behaviors*.

FRUSTRATIONS IN LEARNING

Learning not only puzzles students on occasion, but teachers as well. Consider the following commentary from a literature professor:

"If you reach 10 percent of your students, you're a good teacher." In 13 years as a college English teacher, I've heard that too often. Can you imagine your mechanic saying, "If I fix 10 percent of the cars in my shop, I'm a good mechanic"? Or your doctor: "If I heal 10 percent of my patients, I'm a good doctor"? That's a 90 percent kill rate.

For many of my teaching years, I had a 90 percent kill rate. I'd been talking my students to death. It was 1971 when it hit me. I was lecturing to my American literature class about Henry James. After class a student came to me and said, "Something you said I didn't get down right. Would you repeat it for me please? I'm student teaching in the fall and I want to give this stuff to my high school lit class." I was stunned. This young man wanted to present my words and ideas to his students. He felt no need to stir my lecture into his own understanding. He felt no need to consider what high schoolers would respond to. He would just lecture them my lecture. Where had he gotten such ideas?

Obviously, from me. From all his teachers.

That student confirmed my suspicions about myself and most of my university teachers. We are teaching badly. Horribly, in fact. For me that day in 1971 started an anxious search. There had to be a better way. Since then I've come to some firm answers about these old questions. What is learning? When and how do people learn?

When and how did I learn? I sometimes ride a bike to school. When I think back to how I learned to ride, I remember a heavy green and white girl's bike from Sears. I was seven, the youngest in my family, and too small to reach the pedals on my brother's bike. My dad's store, with candy, cookies, and all that, was three blocks away. I went there several times a day, and I was tired of walking. Besides, smaller kids than I could ride two-wheelers.

I straddled the bike and came down hard on the top pedal. I tipped over. I got back on and tipped again. The bike pinned me under and I scraped a thigh on the sidewalk. But I had to learn, so I kept at it. In a week I could ride pretty well. Today I can also read, write, ski, and even fix the clothes dryer in my home. I learned them all the same way.

There is something so simple, so universal in this learning pattern. I needed to know or do something, so I went after it. It was hard and hurt sometimes, but it worked. But when I think about what I learned in classrooms, that bike-riding pattern seldom happened. Often I sat passive, waiting for class to be over.

(From Kraft, R. G. Bike riding and the art of learning. *Change,* 1978, 10, 38–42.)

What kind of teacher will you be? The challenge will be to stimulate students in the gymnasium or classroom as they are motivated to play outside of school.

Educational psychologists have conveniently categorized learning activities as being primarily *psychomotor* (another name for *motor*), *cognitive,* or *affective.* As we can see in Figure 1–1, behaviors can be and have been classified rather conveniently as to primary activities: the psychomotor *(to do);* the cognitive *(to know);* and the affective *(to feel).* Many approaches to the analysis of behaviors have been offered. Figure 1–2 contains another perspective, as suggested by Robert Gagné (1977). Although differences can be noted among various approaches to classification, motor skills typically are isolated as a unique area of consideration. In other words, special recognition is given to motor skills, with implications for instruction.

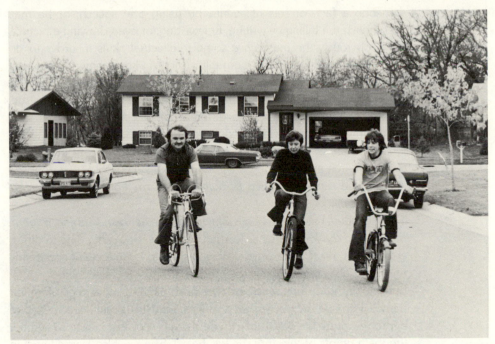

Featherkill Studios

Bicycling: easily learned and well-remembered.

VARIETIES OF LEARNING

Figure 1–2 represents, according to Gagné, five major categories of human performance that may be established by learning. He describes them as follows:

1. An individual may learn to interact with the environment by *using symbols*. As a child, she uses oral language to deal with her environment symbolically, as when she says "Open!" as a request to her parent to open a door, or as a response to such a parental request. Reading and writing and using numbers are basic kinds of symbol use learned in early grades. As the learning of school subjects continues, symbols are used in more complex ways: distinguishing, combining, tabulating, classifying, analyzing, and quantifying objects, events, and even other symbols. Mentally translating 24 ounces into pounds is a simple example; making a singular verb agree with a singular subject in a written sentence is another. This kind of learned capability is given the name *intellectual skill*.

2. A person may learn to *state* or *tell* some information. He may tell

someone a fact, or sets of events, by using oral speech; or he may accomplish the telling by writing, typewriting, or even drawing a picture. Now, obviously, he must *have* some intellectual skills in order to do this stating. In other words, he must ordinarily know how to construct at least simple sentences. But the purpose of the learner's act is to *tell information,* not to display the intellectual skill of sentence construction. The stating done by two different people may vary in its skill, yet the information (the ideas) conveyed may be indistinguishable. What is stated may be a single idea, or a set of ideas which are ordered in some way (as in recounting a set of events). Being able to state ideas is a learned capability called *verbalizable information,* or simply *verbal information.*

3. The individual has learned *skills which manage her own learning, remembering, and thinking.* She has learned certain ways of attending to different parts of a text, for example. When asked to learn a set of apparently unrelated object-names, she approaches the task by searching for relationships among the names, or relationships with other more familiar names. Perhaps the learner has acquired a particular skill which enables her to recapture the details of a scene she has witnessed, or to remember the main points of a lecture she has heard. She has also learned certain techniques of thinking, ways of analyzing problems, approaches to the solving of problems. These skills, which control the learner's own internal processes are given the general name of *cognitive strategies.*

4. The human learner has learned to *execute movements* in a number of organized motor acts, as in threading a needle or throwing a ball. Often these individually coherent acts form a part of more comprehensive activities such as playing tennis or driving an automobile. The unitary acts are reffered to as *motor skills.*

5. The learner has acquired mental states which *influence his choices of personal actions.* He may tend to choose actions that increase the likelihood of his choosing golf, for example, as a preferred recreation. Or he may choose to study physics rather than English literature during the time available for study. Such "tendencies," which are observed as *choices* on the part of the learner, rather than as specific performances, are called *attitudes.*

Here, then, are the five major categories of capabilities that human beings learn. These categories are intended to be comprehensive. Any learned capability, regardless of how it is otherwise described (as mathematics, history, economics, or whatever), has the characteristics of one or another of these varieties.

(From Gagné, R. M. *The Conditions of Learning,* third edition. New York: Holt, Rinehart and Winston, 1977, pp. 27–28

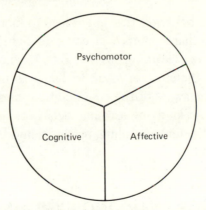

Figure 1–1. Three ways of classifying behaviors from an educational psychology point of view.

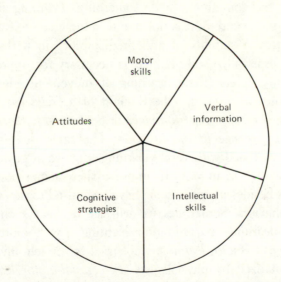

Figure 1–2. Another perspective in the classifications of behaviors.

Experimental psychologists have tended to dissect behaviors differently, sometimes distinguishing among such learnings as motor learning, perceptual learning, problem-solving, probability learning, and others. It is probably true that there are unique considerations for different types of learning, although there is no agreement as to how many types there are. Yet there are many commonalities among the different kinds of learning.

In dealing with motor skills, it is often difficult to separate types of behavior involved in learning and performance, since all together contribute to level of skill. In fact, the sensitive teacher is always on the lookout for ways to improve the operation of all those behaviors that might lead to more meaningful learning.

As we proceed, perhaps points will come to light where commonalities appear across various types of learnings, as well as factors unique to motor learning and performance. It is therefore of value to know as much as we can about learning in general, to be aware of the considerations and conditions that seem to be operative for most kinds of learning behaviors as well as about those that apply especially to the understanding, teaching, and learning of motor skills.

MOTOR LEARNING EXPLAINED

Learning suggests that a change occurs. This change occurs in one's ability to know something, feel something, or do something. *Learning* also suggests that whatever change has occurred, it is not due to some chance. Rather, with more learning comes greater stability of and predictability in performance. Consequently practice, especially good practice, is necessary for improvement.

Motor learning refers to the learning of movement-oriented skills. And by definition, motor learning may be thought of as *reflected or inferred by a relatively permanent change in performance or behavioral potential resulting from practice or past experience in the situation.* The same definition would hold true if we were concerned with verbal learning. But we are interested in motor behaviors here, as well as in ways to improve their acquisition and retention.

Other terms besides *motor learning* have been used to describe the learning of movement behaviors. Sometimes we will see or hear such descriptions as perceptual-motor learning, sensori-motor learning, psychomotor learning, and motor control. *Sensori-motor learning* is not used too much any more, although it has been popularized by physiologists. *Perceptual-motor learning* is a term favored quite a bit by developmental psychologists or others working with young people. The term *psychomotor learning* has been used to a great extent by educational psychologists.

The term *motor control* has become increasingly popular in recent years. At one time *motor learning* and *motor control* were sort of grouped together and used interchangeably as expressive terms. Now it seems that *motor learning* is concerned more with conditions that are related to improvement in learning (and motor performance), while *motor control* seems to be associated more with internal processes that operate under specified performance conditions.

Motor development and *sport psychology* are currently expanding fields of study, and are quite related to motor learning. Although concerned with all

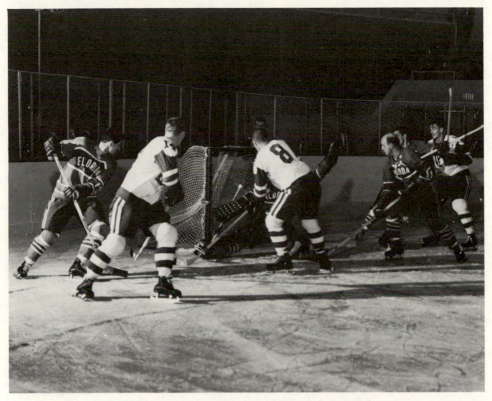

City News Bureau Photo, St. Petersburg, Florida

Skill, physical conditioning, and teamwork in motor performance.

aspects of the developing and maturing organism, motor development specialists typically focus on how children learn and on the conditions that will improve their learning. Sport psychology targets in on athletes and those who participate in sports activities. It addresses personal and personality factors, group dynamics, psychometrics, and the acquisition and maintenance of skill. Evidently, motor learning is of interest in both motor development and sport psychology.

As we read and analyze the published literature, we find varying terms used to describe similar phenomena associated with learning. The varied terms represent the backgrounds and interests of variously trained scholars and how they prefer to explain their research. This situation can be confusing, and so Figure 1–3 is offered for clarification. An understanding and recognition of such terms will make it easier to interpret the research literature and the meaning of experimental findings.

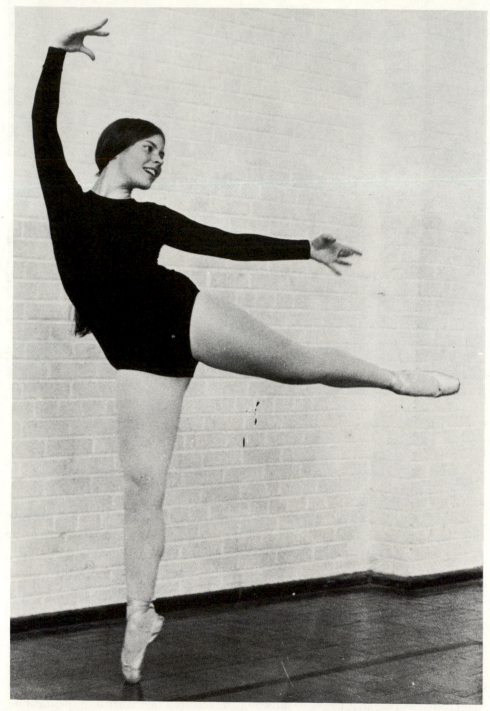

Featherkill Studios, Burnsville, MN

The aesthetics of motor skill.

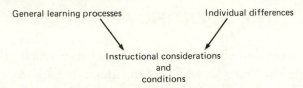

Figure 1–3. An understanding of similarities and differences among learners leads to improved instructional considerations and conditions.

BEHAVIORAL TERMS AND LEARNING

Different terms are used to describe similar phenomena, according to different theories or models.

Theory or Model	Situation	Activity
behavioristic	stimulus	response
systems	input	output
information processing	information	behavior
performance	cue, signal	performance

(From Singer, R. N. *Motor Learning and Human Performance*, third edition. New York: Macmillan, 1980.

The terms are associated with the process and observation of learning. Any situation has the potential to cause a person to react to it. Motor learning involves the developing ability to execute an appropriate movement in achieving a goal.

To what do we respond? Researchers have used such terms as *stimulus, input, signal, information,* and *cues* interchangeably, depending on their theoretical orientations. The act has been termed a *response, output, behavior,* or *performance.* As you read Chapter 2 on theories, these terms will reappear in theoretical contexts. However, many of these terms are referred to in everyday language anyway. Even such expressions as *input* and *output* are more common as computers and computer language become more familiar to us.

These terms will be elaborated upon later, but for now, you are at least prepared for terms used in the research literature that bear on learning and performance. Study them carefully. A knowledge of them will help you to read diverse articles on motor learning, and to make sense of them.

THE SCIENTIFIC APPROACH

The study of learning and ultimate decisions about instruction can either reflect best guesses or derive from scientific information. Researcher-scientists implement a *scientific approach* (or *method*) in conducting research. In other words, a formalized, systematic, organized process is used in the collection of data: information of interest, observations of behavior. We can therefore expect that the information derived from this process is reasonably accurate and helpful. When research findings are in agreement, we can confidently hold a belief about some aspect of learning.

Many books contain information dealing with scientific methods in research. At various levels of sophistication, such resources are potentially helpful to beginning or more expert researchers. It would benefit you to become acquainted with research procedures and statistics to some degree, in order to be able to more fully comprehend, analyze, and interpret the results of investigations. Without this background, you will have to rely on the interpretations that others make of research findings (as I and others do in textbooks of this sort). Textbooks are good first steps in becoming familiar with an area, but by necessity they are typically quite general. But a reading of an introductory book should start you off in the right direction. Even if you don't possess a researcher's professional tools now, maybe you will later.

Research strategies may go in various directions, depending on the purpose of the research and behaviors of interest. Most of the research on learning, at least in this country, has been *experimental* in nature. That is to say, *variables* are *controlled* and one variable may be *manipulated* to determine *cause and effect*. That is, if something is added to, subtracted from, or modified in a situation, what will be the consequences? For example, if videotape is added to an instructional program in gymnastics, will students learn more than when no videotape is used? When reward and punishment situations are compared in a tennis class, which will lead to better learning?

Questions like these are endless. Experimental research can help provide answers to them. Experimental evidence allows one to predict outcomes in future situations when certain factors are present. For instance, on the basis of evidence we may usually expect that people who establish high, specific, but attainable goals in a learning/performance situation will fare better than those who do not. From an instructional perspective, the implication would be that students should be helped to establish such goals.

Besides experimental research, *descriptive research* also provides valuable insights into questions associated with learning. Whereas experimental research describes what *will be* (that is, it is predictive), descriptive research reveals what *is*. Relationships between factors are established. Will those who achieve well in a basketball class do the same in a volleyball class? Will the kids in a third-grade class who tend to perform at a higher level than their classmates be stronger and larger than they are? Descriptive research does not indicate cause and effect, but rather the degree to which at least two variables are related, or go together.

Motor learning research has been primarily oriented toward experimental methods and secondarily toward descriptive methods. The information derived from both approaches is of considerable value in contributing to the body of knowledge about motor learning.

RESEARCH

Information that aids us in making appropriate decisions about these areas can be gained from past experience, advice given by respected others, and research findings. It is the last source that is of primary concern here. For approximately one hundred years now, scholars dedicated to the study of learning have been generating research that should have some bearing on our understanding of learning and ways of improving instruction. Studies have been conducted in laboratory as well as real-world settings. Humans as well as animals have been used as subjects. *Laboratory settings* allow for a greater control over subjects and conditions, but there typically is a great deal of artificiality associated with laboratory research. On the other hand, *real-world research*, such as that conducted in classrooms, gymnasiums, pools, and athletic fields, tends to bring the research closer to where the real interest may be. But there is great difficulty in controlling aspects of real-world study, and in collecting data as sensitive and precise as might be collected in a laboratory setting.

Both types of research are important and necessary. Typically, problems identified in everyday life are recognized and studied under carefully controlled laboratory settings. When the findings resulting from such laboratory studies are of a meaningful nature and point in a particular direction, they generate ideas for practical applications as well as for research that might be conducted in real-life settings. Ideally, research in real settings would confirm the laboratory research findings. Of course, there are times when people undertake practical research for the sake of making applications in an immediate context; this is called *applied* or *action research*. Likewise, there are scholars who undertake research to contribute to a body of knowledge and to conceptual directions; this type of research is considered *basic* or *pure*. Regardless of intention, both types can and do make meaningful contributions to the understanding of the learner and of learning processes and conditions.

MAJOR CONSIDERATIONS IN MOTOR LEARNING

Although there are many, many considerations that we should bear in mind in trying to understand how people learn skills and can learn them best, they can be categorized (see Figure 1–3) into three major areas:

(1) Learning and performance processes (processes that seem to work the same for most people).

(2) Individual differences (ways in which people seem to differ in terms of how they learn and respond to situations).

(3) Instructional conditions (ways in which to manipulate learning environments or tasks in order to faciliate learning for people in general or with respect to individual differences).

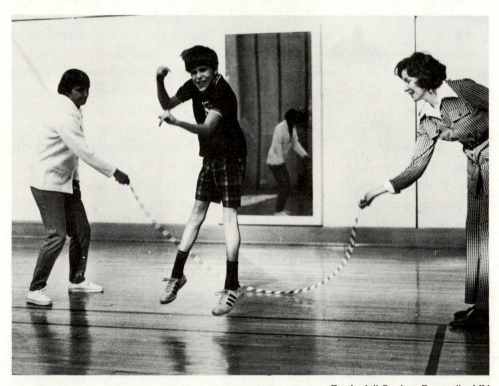

Featherkill Studios, Burnsville, MN

Motor activity for the mentally retarded.

By *learning processes* we mean the kinds of activities that people undergo when they notice that there is something in a situation to which they are supposed to respond. The movement of a ball which is to be caught or hit must be anticipated. The water and its characteristics must be observed before jumping or diving into it in order to swim. Such preparatory activites lead to the processing of information. When we observe situations and interpret them, the next step is usually to make some decision as to what to do in them. A plan of action is decided upon, and movement may be generated. Once the movement is generated, there may be some information available to the person as to how he or she is doing during performance or after it. This generalized sequence of events, from the time the information is received to the time that the performance is effected and we are aware of how we are doing or how we have just done, suggests that people tend to use similar processes as they learn and perform skills.

Since there are obvious differences in the way performances occur from person to person, some people evidently use processes more effectively than others. Skill differences are due to other factors as well. Later, we will analyze

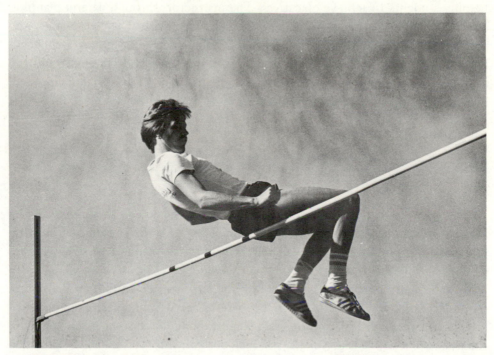

Featherkill Studios, Burnsville, MN

A motor skill involving power.

in more depth the kind of processes that most people apply to learning and performance situations in which motor skills are involved.

With respect to *individual differences,* a number of factors contribute to differential influences on learning and performance in a somewhat predictable manner. Performances may vary among people due to level of motivation, attitudes, reactions to anxiety, age, prior experiences, abilities, and numerous other factors. As teachers and coaches, most of the time we attempt to communicate with students and athletes in a group situation. In other words, instruction is delivered in such a manner as to be effective with the average member of the group. It is preferable when, in addition to this type of instruction, there is the possibility for special treatment to be given to those individuals who are not responding desirably to the standard approach. There are great differences in the way people learn and how much they learn. First we need to understand those major factors that tend to differentiate people in learning and performance; the next step is to determine what to do about such differences when they are found to exist.

Once we have understood learning processes in general, and have identified the ways in which individuals may differ in a meaningful manner, the next step is to develop *instructional conditions and plans* that are most effective in helping students to achieve objectives. The instructor, through careful planning and the design of instruction, will have much to do with what what is learned and how well it is learned. An awareness of such factors as motivational techniques, communication styles, the use of reinforcement and feedback, and the application of media and specialized equipment, and many other factors will help to improve instructional conditions.

THE SCOPE OF THIS BOOK

As has been indicated, the primary purpose of this book is to summarize the available research and to show how to apply it to our understanding of learning processes and conditions. We will rely heavily on scientific evidence, whether it comes from the laboratory or from real-world conditions. We will need to deal with theory to some degree in order to gain a better handle on the nature of motor skills and how they can be best learned. In addition, in order to understand research on learning, it is important to have some background in the nature of learning experiments and their designs. Information will be provided on topics related to experimentation and the measurement of learning.

Following this, motor learning tasks will be categorized in various ways, to indicate how they have been categorized and the reasons for such procedures. Classification systems can be of value, as we will see. Analyzed will be the acquisition of skill; that is, how people learn. Personal factors will be identified. Practice conditions will also be examined, as they can influence the way people acquire skills.

With quality practice and appropriate motivation, skill should increase When we say that someone is *highly skilled,* what in fact do we mean? How do the learning/performance processes of the highly skilled operate? How are they different in comparison to those of the less skilled? Characteristics of skilled behavior will be discussed. Motor learning will be explained in terms of its implications for physical education and sports programs. Finally, learning principles based on the evidence provided in this book will be presented in outline form. In essence, this outline will summarize the content of this entire book.

SUMMARY

In this introductory material, the intention was to give you some feeling for what is meant by the term *motor learning,* and what the major considerations are in this area. Cognitive, affective, and motor behaviors were discussed with the aim of providing a framework for the understanding of motor learning. The primary considerations in motor learning are learning processes, individual differences, and instructional conditions. The understanding of these three areas from a scientific perspective, as well as ways to use that information to aid learners, should be your ultimate goal.

REFERENCES AND SUGGESTED READINGS

References will be suggested at the end of each chapter in case you would care to read any further on the topics covered.

Gagné, R. M. *The conditions of learning,* third edition. New York: Holt, Rhinehart and Winston, 1977, Chapter 2.

Melton, A. W. (ed.) *Categories of human learning.* New York: Academic Press, 1964.

Singer, R. N. *Motor learning and human performance,* third edition. New York: Macmillan Publishing Co., Inc., 1980, Chapter 1.

Singer, R. N. (ed.) *The psychomotor domain: movement behaviors.* Philadelphia: Lea & Febiger, 1972.

2

DIRECTIONS
IN
RESEARCH
AND THEORY

It has been stated that one of the most important considerations in the study of learning is the nature of those processes that people use in general as they learn and perform skills. What will most people think about and how will they react in the same learning situation? What are those processes that any of us might activate in order to acquire a skill? Individuals differ in a number of ways, but there are ways in which most of us will behave alike, given the same circumstances. This sameness of behavior can be predicted to an extent.

Theories are usually developed in order to describe the way the "average" person might behave in a set of circumstances. Many theories go beyond mere description; indeed, there may be an attempt to predict behavior, given known factors. In this section we will be concerned with the nature of theories of learning and performance, how they are developed and how they can be used. Following a discussion on the nature of theories, you will be introduced to alternative theoretical approaches with special relevance to motor skills and physical education. It will be impossible here to discuss all of the conceptual advancements in the study of behavior. Therefore, only the leading efforts will be presented and highlighted.

THE USE OF RESEARCH AND THEORY

Formalized research associated with learning probably began with the work of the famous German psychologist Ebbinghaus in 1885. Ebbinghaus was very much interested in how people acquire and retain nonsense syllables. Actually, he was really more concerned with the way people learned "real" verbal material, but found it much more convenient to use lists of nonsense syllables in his research. This was because nonsense syllables are unique to people who serve as subjects in an experiment. Since they have not been previously familiarized with such nonsense syllables, all subjects are considered to be beginners, thus they begin practice on an equal basis. In this way, the research can see how long it takes them to learn to some criterion of mastery, as well as how well the learned material is retained over a period of time.

By the way, a nonsense syllable consists of a vowel between two consonants, such as *boq*, *hez*, or *cax*. It is created so as to have no accepted meaning in any language known to the subject. Nonsense syllables have been very popular with psychologists who want to study verbal materials. Likewise "nonsense" tasks have been designed for the study of motor skills. These will be touched upon later. The reason for using "nonsense" tasks in the study of verbal or motor skills, as we mentioned before, is that such activities have not been experienced before by subjects and therefore it is easy to determine cause and effect associations; mainly, to observe the effect of some experimental manipulation on the learning of a task where there has been no previous experience that might contaminate the findings.

Speaking of Ebbinghaus, this is a good opportunity to present performance data in the form of an illustration. Figure 2–1 contains data collected by him on himself. He served as his own subject. It wasn't unheard of in the early days of learning research for experimenters to be their own subjects, and for only one subject to be used in a study. Nowadays, it is unusual for this method to be used, and typically data are collected on a number of subjects. In this way, data can be averaged to rule out the possibility of one person's score or scores being idiosyncratic.

Figure 2–1 demonstrates what happens after something (in this case nonsense syllables) is learned to a criterion of mastery. Ebbinghaus repeatedly tested himself, from 19 minutes afterwards to 31 days later. Fifty-eight per cent of the material was remembered at the first testing point. Twenty-one per cent was recalled after thirty-one days. Research undertaken since that time has revealed similar outcomes: most rapid declines occur right after practice stops, and declines are slower over time. The nature of retention, and how to improve it, will be discussed later.

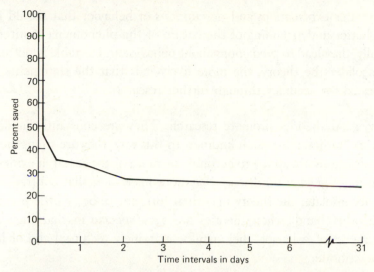

Figure 2–1. Retention of verbal material: The famous Ebbinghaus curve of retention. (From Ebbinghaus, H. *Das Gedächtnis: Untersuchungen zur experimentellen Psychologie.* Leipzig: Duncker and Humblot, 1885.) (Trans. as *Memory: a contribution to experimental psychology* by H. A. Ruger and E. E. Bussenius. New York: Teachers College, Columbia University, 1913).

Since those years in the late 1800s, researchers have developed more refined techniques in the study of learning and behavior. Many types of tasks have been used, and experimental designs have become much more sophisticated. As more and more research accumulates, it is important that an attempt be made to synthesize the findings; they need to be pulled together. Otherwise, there will be only a hodge-podge of fragmented evidence in many different sources, little of which would be of any theoretical value or of practical value. The attempt to bring together research findings in an umbrella fashion, if done scientifically, leads to the formulation of a theory.

Purposes

Theories can have at least four primary characteristics:

(1) They are the result of *facts* and perceptive *analysis* and *synthesis;* they represent the results of one or more researchers who attempt to summarize and to conclude from existing data.

(2) They are usually based on the *law of parsimony*. That is, they tend to explain many facts or observations as briefly as possible.

(3) They offer *explanations* and *descriptions* of behavior that should lead to a better understanding of the nature of the phenomena of interest.

(4) Finally, they lead to *predictions* about behavior and testable hypotheses. The solider the theory, the more likely it is that the statements can be tested for accuracy through further research.

In reality, good theories promote research. They are constantly modified on the basis of contradictory research findings. In this way, they are strengthened as special considerations are added to account for more of the research evidence. Obviously, the more *general* the theory the more likely it is that contradictory evidence may accumulate; the theory may then turn out to be of little practical value. On the other hand, when theories are very *specific* in that they deal with only one aspect of behavior, they may be extremely technical and of little value to the practitioner.

Perspectives

Theories of learning and performance, the concern here, contribute to an understanding of behavior. But so do theories of motivation, thinking, personality, growth and development, group dynamics, etc. Space limitations do not permit a discussion of those areas, unfortunately. Also, the efforts of neuropsychologists and biochemists, in addition to those of educators and psychologists, are extremely relevant to an increased understanding of the nature of learning. Again, space limitations are a problem for us here. Ultimately, the strongest theory of learning is one that incorporates all sorts of research and represents multidisciplinary evidence.

The content and language of a theory indicates the preferences and orientation of a *theorist*. It is virtually impossible to consider all factors influencing or influenced by learning. Yet concentration upon a particular aspect of learning usually results in the neglect of others. Whatever the direction, theories can be studied (1) from the perspective of adding to a body of knowledge and stimulating research, but also (2) for their implications for the improvement of instruction.

The terms *theories, models,* and *systems* have been used somewhat interchangeably in the literature. They all reflect conceptual developments. But usually *theories* are more broadly based whereas *systems* and *models* tend to refer to more specific features of behavior. For convenience, we will use the terms without distinction. In the following pages, the five theoretical approaches will be discussed that seem to have had the most influence on our understanding of behavior in general and motor skills in particular. They are: behaviorism, Gestaltism, information processing, cybernetics, and hierarchical control. Let us turn to behaviorism first.

BEHAVIORISM

At one time, psychology was a part of philosophy. When the two split, there were many who wanted a focus for psychology that was much more tangible than it had been in years past. Instead of dealing with the mind and the soul, the emphasis of these psychologists would be on observable behaviors made in response to specific stimuli.

Just after the turn of this century, behaviorism, as it was to be called, became the dominant school of thought in psychology in this country. Behaviorism was the earliest formal direction of the psychology of learning in this country, being established in the early 1900s by Watson and Thorndike. The emphasis was on learning environment, and the prediction of the nature of responses to particular stimuli by people in general. It provided a formalized direction for psychology. Behaviorists were concerned with the association of predictable responses to specific stimuli, and therefore, this theory was termed *associationistic* or *bond* theory. It was quite mechanistic in nature; in other words, very little consideration was given to individual differences, emotions, and thought processes. Rather, of concern were behaviors that most people seem to exhibit under specifically established conditions.

This can be seen in Figure 2–2. A situation containing a particular stimulus is apt to produce an expected response after sufficient practice. As people become familar with cue or circumstance, they begin to associate a certain behavior with it. Many aspects of behaviorism are related to sports by John Dickinson (1976); Section Four of his work will be of particular interest to you as it deals with the acquisition of skill.

From the behaviorist approach much has been learned about how practice conditions can be improved to be of value to the average person. The teacher, as controller over the learning situation, can create favorable environments conducive to learning. We will address such considerations in Chapter 6. The appropriate use of cues and reinforcements helps. Behavior can be shaped to teach specific acts, but with little regard for other aspects of the the development of the learner. The student may not learn problem-solving skils under a behavioristic approach. Also, the teacher may not gain in understanding or awareness in regard to his or her personal influence over learning processes and movement activities.

Behaviorism has taken many forms through the years. It is still a very strong force in psychology today. It is little wonder that many instructional approaches evolved from behavioristic theory. In physical education and sport situations, the *drill technique* would be a primary example of behaviorism. The teacher or coach blows a whistle or shouts a cue; the students or athletes are expected to respond together and similarly. Similar skills are developed within the students, and they are supposed to respond in the same way to the same cuing techniques. Certainly this approach has its merits, especially in cases where there are many people to be trained under the guidance of one. It is easier to handle large groups when all members are disciplined to respond in the same way to a particular cue.

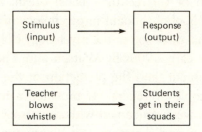

Figure 2–2. The behavioristic approach emphasizes environments and stimuli, and the triggering of associated responses.

Furthermore, many principles related to the use of *rewards and reinforcement* in the shaping of behavior were developed by behaviorists such as the famous Harvard psychologist, B. F. Skinner. He and his colleagues demonstrated how rats and other lower forms of organisms could acquire skills through the use of reinforcements administered intelligently by experimenters. Many instructional and training programs were developed with the same principles in mind, e.g., the use of reinforcements. Reinforcements are inputs that inform a person that he or she is performing in an appropriate manner, and when interjected appropriately by a teacher or coach, they can have a great deal of impact on learning and performance situations. Many reinforcements, such as praise, not only are informational-directive, but they may also help to provide motivation to continue with purpose and inspiration.

Although many basic tenets of behaviorism have prevailed over time, other theoretical approaches have served to weaken certain foundations of it. One of these was the Gestalt school of thought, which was developed in opposition to behaviorism. Let us now turn attention to the beliefs of Gestaltists.

GESTALTISM

Gestaltism developed as an alternative to behaviorism. Whereas behaviorists (associationists) were primarily concerned with the environment and its influence on behaviors, Gestaltists stressed the importance of an *individual's interpretation of the environment*. In other words, Gestaltists were interested in problem-solving, perception, and other processes that individuals use in order to develop appropriate behaviors in response to situations.

In many ways, the Gestalt movement, which primarily took hold in this country during the early 1930s, was the forerunner of what today is called *cognitive psychology*. Cognitive psychology is a very dominant force in psychology at the present time. The development of this concept, in which *thought* and *personal internal organizational* processes are studied and viewed as extremely important in the understanding of learning, can probably be directly associated with those earlier years in which Gestaltists made their contributions. Gestaltists warned us against a doctrine of belief in which humans would be studied and treated as if they were lower forms of organism, reacting in a reflexive manner to various kinds of stimuli. Although behaviorists have contributed much to our understanding of the control and direction of behavior through clever environmental manipulations, the Gestaltists stressed the importance of recognizing individuals as individuals, as well as the particular perceptual processes that they use in order to make meaning of their environments.

All people do not respond similarly in the same situation. Due to genetic differences as well as past differences in experiences, we may not use strategies and processes in the same way in order to achieve the same level of skill. In a sense, then, we must respect the notion that people will and indeed do exhibit different behaviors under similar circumstances on many occasions. Attempts have been made in education to use alternative approaches in helping people to come closer to achieving their maximum potential.

To summarize in a very brief and succinct way the differences between behaviorists and Gestaltists and the implications of their contributions, we have learned from the former about techniques that can be used in learning situations that will have the most profitable impact upon the average learner, and from the latter about ways in which individuals might differ in how they approach a learning situation, and what can be done with them to assist their development. Gestalt and behavioristic theories represent early attempts to study behavior in a scientific manner. In later years, different approaches were developed, primarily due to the fantastic technological advancements that were made during the 1940s. Such developments as the creation of the computer led to new ways of looking at human beings and the study of their behavior.

INFORMATION PROCESSING

Physical educators often only observe behavior itself, with little consideration of those personal processes that influence it. We think in terms of analyzing the response; for instance, whether the basket was made or not, or whether the arrow went into the target. But we rarely think of the way people in general can process information, and the ways that individuals differ due to past experiences, developed capabilities, and any handicap in their systems (visual, auditory, learning disorders, and the like). In information processing theory, the emphasis is on input (sense reception), the transmission of information, and essential central nervous system activities related to decision-making and plans for action.

At one time, information theory was concerned with uncertainty and information, in that information helps to reduce uncertainty. Probability theory was applied to an analysis of situations as to how much information would be needed to resolve a particular dilemma. Through the years a more global perspective has evolved, and now the study of mental capabilities and processes that work on information is associated with information processing theory. In fact, this is the current thrust in cognitive psychology. Much research is being undertaken in regard to the way people receive information, attend to it, organize it, manage it, use memory processes, and ultimately derive a plan of action.

Information processing theory stresses the role of perception, attention, memory, and decision-making. There is a great deal of consideration as to the channel capacity of a person. Borrowed from computer language, *channel capacity* refers to the amount of information that one can handle. How much information can be dealt with at one time? When is the human system being overloaded? When is it underloaded? When is the system being fatigued so that true capacity cannot be demonstrated? How can information be made most accessible in regard to the capacity of a person? What is known about attention? How do learners selectively discriminate among available information? How can they be assisted to discriminate more effectively so that their responses will be most appropriate?

It is not fashionable today to think in terms of specific responses to specific cues, in the old behavioristic framework. Rather, those who are more humanistically oriented like to think of students as information processors, as organisms in the critical stage of developing plans or programs in order to resolve situations. The quality of learning experiences, the type of guidance given for problem-solving, and the emphasis on effective plans of action are considerations the teacher must make and allow for if the child is to develop skills. Likewise, the student needs to learn how to use corrective processes to detect errors in performance and to regulate personal behavior. As we can see, sensory, perceptual,

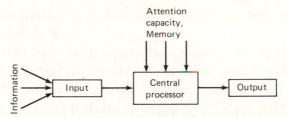

Figure 2–3. The information processing model approach calls to our attention the kinds of processes that are internally activated to organize information, leading to appropriate decisions and effective movements.

decision-making, and output processes all must work together if skilled movement is to be realized. The effective teacher will take special note of the importance of *all* aspects of the human system that contribute to skilled performance.

As Fitts (1964) puts it, "Thus skilled perceptual-motor performance can be viewed as involving operations such as information translation, information transmission, information reduction, information collation, and in some cases the generation of movement. . . . Information storage (memory) is also involved of course" (p. 248). Many models of information processing have been developed. A very basic approach is demonstrated in Figure 2–3. It shows the main subsystems of consideration. *Input* refers to information that comes to the senses (e.g., visual, auditory, kinesthetic information). Essential processing activities are those that occur within the central nervous system. *Output* refers to decision-making that leads to the activation of a pattern of impulses that will in turn innervate particular muscles of the body in order for appropriate movement behavior to occur. An elaboration of the information processing approach is offered by Ronald Martiniuk (1976), with special considerations for physical educators. Many processes and activities occur within a person and ultimately bear on the type of behavior witnessed. Information processing theory is in many ways related to cybernetic theory, to which we will now turn.

CYBERNETICS

Both information processing theory and cybernetic theory were initiated after World War II. The language and ideas of these approaches reflect "the machine age." With the development of advanced and sophisticated equipment, such as computers, new ways were created to analyze human behavior. One of the highlights of cybernetics is the role of *feedback, self-regulation* and *self-monitoring,* techniques that the learner can use in order to help guide learning and to improve skill.

If you recall your beginning psychology classes, discussion invariably centered around S–R concepts (behavioristic theory). As you now know, a stimulus was believed to become conditioned to a particular response, and the learner presumably had little control over this situation. If there is one thing that cybernetic theory has shown us, it is that there is a great deal of control that individual learners can exert over circumstances; many ways in which they can monitor and regulate their own activity. With the acquisition of skill, they learn to depend less on external influences and more on internal (or self-) control and regulatory processes.

Cybernetics means *self-guidance* and *control* of one's own behavior. In the cybernetic approach, it is felt that learning is determined by the sensory effects of the movement or stimulation that accompanies a response. In contrast to the behaviorists, cyberneticians do not typically view reinforcement as a necessity for learning to be demonstrated.

The cybernetics model reflects a servomechanism or *closed-loop* consideration in behavior. In a closed-loop system, once output, or a response, is made, internal feedback potential exists to the receptors—the essential processing mechanisms—as well as to the effectors. This is reflected in Figure 2–4. It is as if the human being can be a self-controlled device with little need for outside intervening controls. In contrast to such a self-governing system, behavioristic theory is *open-loop* in nature. Open-loop systems are limited to reactions that are direct functions of external control, that is, conditions not influenced by internal feedback regulations. Cyberneticians, such as K. U. Smith and Harvey Sussman (1969) believe that the efficiency of performance and the effectiveness of learning depend on properties of the feedback control process.

With development of a skill, people learn how and when to use feedback. During an activity, feedback information may be abundant, redundant, or relatively absent. Consequently, strategies for the use of feedback are important. Feedback can come from the situation or from within the person; it may be

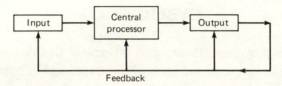

Figure 2–4. The cybernetics model approach emphasizes the role of feedback in the control of ongoing activity. If the act is terminated, feedback information can be stored in memory for future usages.

useful during performance or for subsequent activity if stored as a reference base.

HIERARCHICAL CONTROL

As is the case with information processing and cybernetics models, in adaptive models a comparison is made of a person to a computer. However, the emphases differ with each approach. Your attention was directed in the section on the information processing model to the variation in the capacity of a person to receive and transmit situational information and evolve decisions based on a series of sequential processes. The cybernetic approach emphasizes the roles and uses of feedback control and regulation of movement. The *adaptive* or *hierarchical control model* stresses the role of central processes in controlling and directing movement. Fitts (1964) pointed out similarities and differences among information processing, cybernetic, and hierarchical control models.

In hierarchical control models, *programs* (plans of action) are thought to carry out basic or routine functions in humans as well as in computers. Such basic programs are termed *lower-order programs;* these can be combined to produce more complex or higher-order programs. Higher-level programs can modify lower-order ones on the basis of experience and stored information. Miller, Galanter, and Pribram (1960), in a classic book, made this point very well with regard to human behavior. People's control levels change as their skill is increased. In other words, the beginner will have to conceptualize some sort of movement plan and there will be certain kinds of lower-order programs that need to be executed if his or her higher-order plan is to be fulfilled. As people become more skilled, they are capable of trying to create an image or movement plan of a higher order. This process of selecting routines will improve as skill is increased. With adaptive models, there is concern for the notion of the *relationship of higher order and lower order plans.* This consideration has been most helpful for us in understanding the nature of skilled performance (see Figure 2–5).

How do people tend to perform ongoing acts while still being able to think ahead of strategies and tactics? The basketball player who dribbles the basketball while seemingly paying no attention to it is thinking ahead about uncertain circumstances. With less attention necessary for the ongoing activity, cerebral processes are freed to think ahead, to anticipate. Adaptive models provide us with much useful information with regard to the analysis of behavior, especially as we proceed from lower-order to higher-order behaviors.

Another example may be found in tennis. A high-order program (executive)

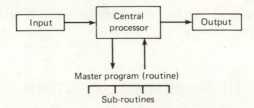

Figure 2–5. The hierarchical control model approach describes central control properties, with master, or executor, routines, and sub-routines. Behavioral control is expressed in a hierarchical fashion: as skill increases, the type and level of control changes.

may be described as "serve and rush to the net," and obviously this complete program would be demonstrated by a higher-skilled performer. The beginning tennis player is panicked about merely throwing the ball up straight in the air and he or she prays that ball contact is good, let alone worrying about rushing to the net. The highly skilled performer is able to implement a complex movement plan for not only hitting the ball and hitting it into the court correctly, but rushing to the net simultaneously as well. These, of course, are the independent lower-order kinds of behaviors that need to be learned first if the executive plan is going to be realized. Task analysis and person (level of skill) analysis would suggest the appropriate executive program that needs to be conceptualized and developed.

INTEGRATING THE CONCEPTS

Each of the contemporary models discussed is useful for the student of learning and teacher of skills. An integration of cybernetic, information processing, and adaptive models is a logical approach to identify the most important processes and mechanisms in the human behaving system, how they are related, and how they function to determine learning and performance. By understanding how people are similar in their behaving and functioning processes (and what may contribute to any differences), instructors, trainers, and coaches can become more effective in developing skills within learners.

IMPLICATIONS FOR TEACHING AND LEARNING MOTOR SKILLS

From what we have covered so far, it can be seen that there is much that can be done by the teacher to influence the achievements of others; and much that can be done by the learners themselves, for themselves. Many specific teaching and learning considerations will be dealt with throughout the book. For now, however, we realize that

(1) learning situations can be arranged in many ways, and scientific evidence indicates those that have the highest probability of influencing people in general to achieve goals effectively;

(2) many internal processes interact to produce learning;

(3) people actively make their own sense of situations, and consequently may behave differently from each other or even within themselves on repeated occasions;

(4) learners need to learn how to manage and process information more effectively, to make their capacities more functional; and

(5) skill is a function of
   a. capabilities related to input (sensory-perceptual activities),
   b. central processing (organization, management, and decision-making), and
   c. output (motor functions and feedback utilization).

On one hand, the teacher can help to shape the behaviors of students by wisely administering cues, reinforcement, and feedback. Practice conditions for the learning of a sports activity can be structured according to (1) the nature of the demands of the activity, (2) the objectives in the situation, and (3) the skill level of the students. And ideas for this structuring can be derived from research in the psychology of learning area.

On the other hand, and in a complementary fashion, the teacher can help learners acquire appropriate strategies that will facilitate the operation of the internal processes associated with their information processing. Such strategies may aid not only in the learning of a skill, but in its retention over time as well. In addition, strategies can influence the transfer of learning—the degree to which the learning of one skill promotes the learning of a related skill. A discussion on the nature of learner strategies and their influence on achievement can be found in Chapter 6.

For those of you interested in a more elaborate understanding of learning theories, their development, nature, and applications, a number of excellent books are available. Hilgard and Bower (1975) provide extraordinary coverage of learning theories within an historical context. A comprehensive treatment of systems and theories, with historical developments, is offered by Chaplin and Krawiec (1974). And Snelbecker's (1974) book is primarily oriented toward the application of theory to instruction; it provides an interface of psychological theory with the concerns of the educator.

The application of behavioral science technology and research to instruction reflects an orderly and systematic attempt to improve instruction. We are encouraged to think more carefully and clearly about the nature of the learning activities and the nature of learners. Research findings dealing with behavior can be translated into more favorable instructional strategies and learning environments in our own teaching situations.

SUMMARY

Research is the scientist's tool to determine the truth, and it is the substantive basis upon which theories are formulated. Theories of learning are based on scientific evidence, describe phenomena of interest, are parsimonious in that they reflect the theorist's ability to synthesize and reduce voluminous material to a more easily comprehensible form, and may have predictive value. Although criticized on occasion for being too far removed from reality, theories in many cases have stimulated research and also given rise to prescriptive decisions made by educators for students.

Theories may be broad-based or developed for the study of a particular concern, such as memory. The language and orientation of theories differ quite a bit, depending on the background of the theorist and his or her purpose. Behaviorism was the earliest formal direction of the psychology of learning in this country, being established in the early 1900s by Watson and Thorndike. The emphasis was on the learning environment, and the prediction of the nature of responses to particular stimuli by people in general. Gestaltists challenged this orientation in the 1930s. They were concerned with perceptions, analysis, problem-solving—how people made sense out of their environments.

The 1940s brought new concepts in viewing behavior. Technology and human behavior were wedded in both conceptual directions and terminology. Three distinct yet related person-machine analogy models were promoted: information processing, cybernetics, and hierarchical control. Although each has been interpreted in various ways, they may be highlighted as follows, with implications for the physical educator.

In information processing models, the emphasis is on the nature of situational information and how and what is received, perceived, attended to, memorized, and used in that situation by a person. In other words, information processing capacities and abilities and ways to improve them are the focal points. The main contribution of cybernetic models is the understanding of the role of feedback in performance monitoring, regulation, and improvement. In many instances we have the ability to use information available to us as a result of our actions to control those movements. Hierarchical control models stress the development of master programs that guide acts. With increased skills, a person uses higher-order programs, or plans, to control lesser-order routines. Table 2–1 highlights the different theories.

_____ **TABLE 2–1** _____

A Comparison of Conceptual Approaches with Implications for Teaching

Theory or Model	Major Emphases	Implications for Teaching
behavioristic approach	nature of the learning environment stimulus-response associations conditioning or shaping behavior	group-centered approach drill or formal teaching techniques use of rewards and other types of reinforcers
Gestalt approach	nature of personal perception of the learning environment thought processes, problem-solving	respect for individual differences structuring learning experiences for problem solving
information processing approach	attentional, memorial, and other internal processes associated with the organization and meaning of information capacities and functioning	concern for the manner in which information is presented organizational techniques to improve the processing of information
cybernetic approach	feedback influence over behavior self-regulation, monitoring, and control	learner's ability to use own self-guidance techniques
hierarchical control approach	central processes and their control over behavior programs, plans, and master routines governing of sub-routines shifting of control	task analysis and teaching at appropriate level for proper skill development determining level of control and one's ability level

REFERENCES AND SUGGESTED READINGS

Chaplin, J. P. and Krawiec, T. S. *Systems and theories of psychology,* third edition. New York: Holt, Rinehart and Winston, 1974.

Dickinson, J. *A behavioral analysis of sport.* Princeton, N.J.: Princeton Book Co., 1976, Section 4.

Fitts, P. M. Perceptual-motor skill learning. In A. W. Melton (ed.), *Categories of human learning.* New York: Academic Press, 1964.

Hilgard, E. R. and Bower, G. H. *Theories of learning,* fourth edition. Englewood Cliffs, N. J.: Prentice-Hall, 1975.

Marteniuk, R. G. *Information processing in motor skills.* New York: Holt, Rinehart and Winston, 1976.

Miller, G. A., Galanter, E., and Pribram, K. H. *Plans and the structure of behavior.* New York: Holt, Rinehart and Winston, 1960.

Singer, R. N. *Motor learning and human performance,* third edition. New York: Macmillan Publishing Co., Inc. 1980, Chapters 4, 5, and 6.

Smith, K. U. and Sussman, H. Cybernetic theory and analysis of motor learning and memory. In E. A. Bilodeau (ed.), *Principles of skill acquisition.* New York: Academic Press, 1969.

Snelbecker, G. E. *Learning theory, instructional theory, and psychoeducational design.* New York: McGraw-Hill, 1974.

3

THE MEASUREMENT

OF LEARNING

So far, some basic concepts about learning have been described. We know it's important to influence learning conditions and processes—to expedite the acquisition and guiding of skill. But how do we know when learning is taking place?

This may seem like a stupid question. But consider the following case. A student is learning to play golf. Scores fluctuate on occasion, but generally work their way down from 128 to 95. Learning definitely seems to be occurring. But then, scores over the next three weeks start getting worse. Is no learning occurring with practice? Is the person learning the wrong things? Or is this merely the process of putting together higher-order strategies and skills, with the inevitable worse scores not truly indicative of what's going on? Sooner or later, once solidified, performance level will more aptly represent learning level.

The importance of being able to *measure learning* is at the heart of determining instructional effectiveness. It is informative (and hopefully motivational) to the learner. For the researcher very sensitive indices of learning are required, as associated with specified conditions, for he or she wants to use statistical probability to determine if and how processes and behaviors are influenced in a meaningful manner. Generalizations may then be made from the findings in scientific investigations to suggest instructional procedures for the gymnasium, athletic field, or pool.

In this chapter, we will explore the relationship between learning and performance. We will discuss learning curves, how they are plotted and averaged, and what they indicate. Some unit of information has to be decided upon to represent the learning score in a situation, and the measure of the learning itself. Alternatives and rationales will be explored. Finally, the nature of learning experiments will be addressed. Sample experiments will be provided to give you a feel of how some basic ideas are put to the test.

LEARNING AND PERFORMANCE

Earlier we identified a problem in golf: does a continual comparison of performance scores by the same person indicate level of learning? Of course, this problem is a problem in every observation and measurement case. How can we assess the learning level of a person?

The answer is that we assess it through some observable behavior, some measure of performance. It's the best procedure we have. Unfortunately, it does not always represent a true level of proficiency, or at least one perceived by the student. How many of you have taken a test in a class and thought you knew better than what you demonstrated? In the past, have you experienced mental lapses? Too much anxiety? Too little motivation? Bad testing procedure? Have you wondered, will the same situation occur in this class??

For the performance measure to come close to reflecting the learning level, both teacher and student, experimenter and subject, have responsibilities. The teacher or experimenter should establish *testing conditions* that are clearly *understood* by all; they must be scientifically *valid* and *reliable*. They must be *consistent* and *fair* from person to person. The student or subject should be adequately *prepared*, psychologically, physically, and cognitively, to be tested. He or she should be prepared not only for the content of the test, but for the process of test-taking as well. In the classroom or in the laboratory, only the most optimal conditions should prevail when people are being evaluated, to maximize the potential matching of test performance level and learning status.

As a final consideration in determining learning through performance, we do not wish to confound our conclusions with other variables. For instance, children may improve in an activity practiced over a long time simply because of *maturational factors*. As the neurological system develops, capabilities improve. In our discussion about learning, we typically try to exclude maturation as a variable that might confuse our understanding of how learning processes operate and the way learning conditions will affect them.

Furthermore, a subject's *health status, personal problems, anxiety, motivation, unfair anticipation of task demands*, or *luck* may produce a performance score quite incompatible with the same subject's theoretical "true" learning status for a given activity. Ideally, testing conditions would be devised to control for these factors as much as possible. In fact, this is one of the reasons why many subjects are used in experiments, and their scores averaged. Extreme high or low individual scores, due to such factors, should thereby contribute a minimal bias to the data. Of course in some studies a number of these factors, such as anxiety or motivation, may be of interest to investigate in and of themselves.

LEARNING SCORES

What type of behavior should be looked at to assess learning? This question may not be as easy as it appears. Let us take a tennis class. We would want to know how much learning has been influenced as a result of our instruction. Should we devise or use an already constructed test or tests to assess individual tennis strokes (e.g., forehand, backhand, serve)? Should we observe the students during practice or competitive conditions, and subjectively evaluate them? Or might we hold a class round-robin tournament to determine the relative standing of each student? Do you favor something else? All of these approaches?

With the laboratory tasks typically used in motor learning experiments, quantitative data such as reaction time and/or movement speed may be of interest. *Accuracy of movement* and/or *speed* are possible sources of data with certain tasks. Even inaccuracy, or *error*, in movement with static or moving targets can be analyzed from different behavioral and mathematical perspectives. Thus we may determine time on target *(TOT)* with movable objects. Under static settings, absolute error *(AE)*, variable error *(VE)*, or constant error *(CE)* may be derived from the same set of data, where

AE = the magnitude of an error in performance, with no indication of the direction of the error relative to the target.

VE = the variability of performance, or conversely, response consistency for a number of trials.

CE = the magnitude of an error in performance with an indication of the direction of the error relative to the target; whereas *AE* provides average error, *CE* indicates response bias

The typical performance measures in motor learning experiments are:

(1) *Reaction time,* which is the time elapsed between the onset of a "go" signal and the initiation of a response.

(2) *Duration of movement* to complete a task or time to complete a movement.

(3) *Accuracy of movement* in relation to a target or criterion.

(4) *Extent of movement outcome,* as to number of correct performances within a time period, number of points scored, height jumped, or number of trials or experiences to reach an established criterion.

In a gymnasium setting, speed and/or accuracy of movement is usually important in physical activities. So is extent of movement outcome. But there are additional considerations. One of the typical techniques in the real world is *subjective evaluation* of form, of playing ability, etc. This approach is rarely used in the laboratory. Another technique is to assess *problem-solving ability*, as in movement education approaches in physical education. There may be *no one correct pre-established* response. Rather, alternative movement possibilities may exist within the situational and personal constraints established by the teacher.

In many educational systems today, teachers have to prespecify the *objectives* of their instruction and how these objectives will be assessed. The objectives of any experiment or class experience should indicate appropriate assessment techniques.

In class or experimental situations, often more than one type of measure can be used as a learning score. So how do we decide how to measure? One of the rules is the law of parsimony: use the least number of measures possible and *avoid redundancy* (useless duplication). Redundancy testing is a waste of time. Another consideration is the *time, human resources*, and *equipment available* for testing. Constraints in these areas may impose limitations on otherwise desirable testing procedures.

In experimental settings, the *learning processes* being assessed may suggest which type of scoring technique is more useful than another. Then too, *different measures may reflect different aspects of learning*, and so all of these may be considered as useful information. For instance, both speed and accuracy are important contributors to success in a number of activities. Perhaps scores for each separately, or combined in some formula, would be an appropriate approach to measuring certain tasks under certain experimental conditions.

Whatever is determined as the data, or information, to be examined, a good rationale for that decision should be constructed. Data should be as accurate as possible, with minimum human or machine error. Information should be comprehensive but not redundant. The type and quality of any learning or achievement score or scores derived in any class or experimental settings will serve as the basis for conclusions about the effectiveness of instruction or a particular experimental condition.

LEARNING MEASURES

An equally relevant decision concerns the procedure to be used to assess achievement. Let's make the issue very simple by example. In your archery class, you administered three similar tests: one at the beginning, one in the middle, and one at the end. What is a fair score to give to the students? Should you average all three, use only the last one, or determine the difference or gains from the first test to the last test?

Averaging scores on tests taken over time or at one time provides you with more information to work from. The process discourages the problem that just one score may bring up—the possible unusually high or low score, not truly indicative of learning status.

On the other hand, merely using a posttest or final test(s) may be what really counts. We may care only about ultimate achievement, not scores along the way. Then again, pre- and posttest comparisons may be of great concern, especially if people have not entered the learning situation with the same level of skill and we would like to determine improvement scores.

Why not discuss the relative values and limitations of each technique: (1) *the average score*, (2) *the final score*, and (3) *the improvement score*. Other considerations can be added to those we have just outlined. What procedure do you favor? Why?

To confuse the matter further, a number of other possibilities are available as well. One of the most frequently used techniques in learning experiments is to administer *repeated tests* under the same conditions to subjects. In that way performances from trial to trial or blocks of trials can be compared: within a group of subjects (change) and between groups of subjects.

A Sample Experiment

Let's work with some data here. Our concern might be to design an experiment to determine the effectiveness of having subjects set specific, high, but attainable goals for themselves. We might hypothesize that these subjects *should* learn and perform better than subjects who are not given such guidance. How will we test this hypothesis?

We might form two groups of subjects. The experimental one is provided with assistance in goal-setting; the control is not. Any performance differences observed will be due to the goal-setting experience, assuming that all *other* factors that might influence the subjects and their learning/performance abilities have been *reasonably controlled*. A learning task must be decided upon: let's say it involves throwing six balls, behind the back, at a target of concentric circles with different values. Points are awarded, depending upon degree of accuracy. Perhaps 15 trials will be administered. The design is as follows:

Groups	Trials														
	1	2	3	4	5	6	7	8	9	10	11	12	13	14	15
Goal-setting group															
Control group															

Performance scores are collected following each trial for each subject in each group. If there were 15 subjects in a group, scores would be averaged, and a value placed in each box. We will draw learning curves instead, using the same values, to illustrate the hypothetical data. By the way, the way such graphics are constructed will be described shortly. Look at Figure 3–1.

Data are plotted for the two groups over 15 trials. Fifty points is the maximum achievement in any trial. What we to know is which group performed (learned) more under the conditions of the study. Visual inspection would lead to an obvious conclusion: goal-setting is more effective than no intention to set goals. But from the researcher's perspective, the data must be analyzed statistically to determine *significant* effects and differences. In other words, are the observations due to chance or are they real? In this sense, "real" means that such differences would occur again, if the same conditions were present. Statistical analysis reveals the probability of such an occurrence.

Let us not worry about types of statistics and how they might be used to analyze the data. What is the appropriate measure to determine the results of the study?

(1) We could average the scores across all the trials for each group. Evidently, the experimental group achieved higher than the control group.

(2) Or, we might only analyze the final scores on trial 15. Again, it looks as though the experimental group was superior.

(3) As to improvement, or gain, scores, it appears that the experimental group learned more than the control group. This observation is made easy as both groups started at approximately the same point. If they had not, it would have been very difficult to evaluate the difference in scores between first and last trials.

(4) But an analysis *during* the learning trials indicates that we can attempt to determine *if* and *when* differences between groups began to occur. From a visual inspection of the scores, there does not appear to be any differences between the groups during the first five trials. Afterwards, the differences become apparent. The goal-setting procedure is more influential after some preliminary practice trials, rather than more effective at each trial. Trial-to-trial analyses or blocks of five trials could be analyzed. *Trend analysis* indicates the points during practice when differences or changes are most significant.

There are many procedural and statistical ways to analyze data. The question must be asked first: What information is most important in the study? Why? Then we can decide on the approach to analyzing the data. If we cared about trends in the data—the possibility that performance goals may not have the same impact at all points in the learning process—the analyses of trials or blocks of trials would be desirable. Then again, if all that we care about is which group achieved the highest level of skill at the end of training, the final scores or trial 15 would be compared between the groups.

Average scores across all trials allow us to determine the general effectiveness of a condition. Gain scores, the difference between last and first scores, provide us with within- and between-group comparisons. For instance, it is possible that both groups improved in a meaningful measure over the course of the

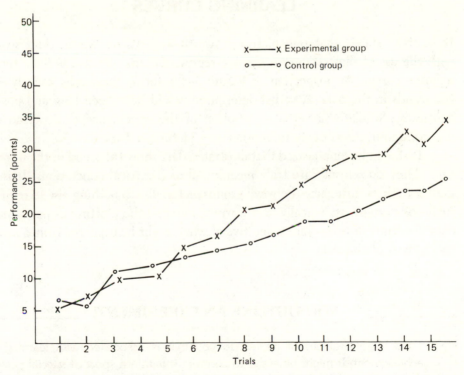

Figure 3–1. Hypothetical data: a comparison of the effectiveness of goal-setting as opposed to no guided goal-setting on learning.

experiment, but the gain of the goal-setting group was higher than that of the control group.

As you can see, various approaches—these and others—are available to the researcher to determine achievement comparisons. Properly controlled experiments allow us to understand more about the nature of learning, which conditions influence it most readily and how they do so. This example experiment should give you a feeling for (1) the identification of a problem worthy of study; (2) a procedure or a plan to evaluate the value of an approach—in this case, goal-setting; (3) how to record and illustrate data; and (4) alternatives in learning measures. But this is but the beginning of our "experimental experience."

Other sample experiments will be presented throughout the book to prod your thinking, to help you create your own investigations of learning phenomena. So will actual research, published in respected scholarly journals. For now, a further analysis of learning curves, experimental procedures, and statistical analyses is in order, and this is the sequence in which the chapter will be concluded.

LEARNING CURVES

It is often stated that one picture is worth a thousand words. And so it is with the use of illustrations, or graphic representations of learning data, termed *learning curves*. An inspection of Figure 3–1 informs the reader quickly as to the trends in the data. A verbal description would have been long and possibly confusing. Similarly, a verbal description of the appearance of a person does not communicate as easily to another as a picture or two.

It should be emphasized that illustrated data show the trend in the information. They *do not* indicate truly meaningful or statistical conclusions. It is one matter to show differences between groups pictorially, something else to reinforce such observations statistically. Yet learning curves—the plotting of performance data over time or trials—are suggestive of what might be expected from a statistical analysis of the data.

YOU OUTLINE AN EXPERIMENT!

Think of a problem of interest to you that is associated with learning and achievement. It might be easier to consider it within a sport of special personal importance. Let's see if you can go through the steps just discussed, using your own writing paper.

(1) *What is the problem?* What will the study determine? Why do you want to do this study? What is its importance? To whom? What will it contribute to?

(2) *What do you hypothesize?* What do you expect to find, and why?

(3) *What is known from the related research?* What do authorities say?

(4) *What is your plan (procedures) to investigate the problem?*

(a) Who are the subjects?

(b) How many groups?

(c) How will the subjects be tested as to any equipment or apparatus? What is their learning task?

(d) What are the procedures *unique* to each group, or at least the experimental group?

(e) What are the procedures in *common* (control factors) for the groups?

(f) What will be your learning score(s)? Why?

(g) How will you assess learning? Why?

(h) Manufacture hypothetical data and plot them in the form of learning curves.

This is far as we need to go. For most of you, a knowledge of statistics will come in a different course, perhaps later in your professional career. Likewise, there is no need here to conclude and imply from your hypothetical data, although you would if working with real data.

Considerations

In a learning curve, a performance measure (a score) is obtained for a subject in each group for each trial, and averaged. Groups can be compared, as was the case in Figure 3–1. Curves can assume many shapes. Some considerations are:

(1) More subjects' scores averaged will tend to smooth the curve; using fewer subjects will lead to irregularities.

(2) More trials averaged, as in blocks of trials, or less trials, will also tend to smooth curves.

(3) The structure, or appearance, of the curve is a function of many variables.

(a) task difficulty.

(b) ceiling effects (the ease in which to achieve maximum performance within the practice time allotted).

(c) the nature of the task and its demands on the learner.

(d) practice conditions.

(e) experimental biasing effects, such as the setting in of fatigue or boredom during the experiment.

Thus, there is no one learning curve. When data are analyzed across subjects, the appearance of the curve will be a function of any one or a combination of the factors mentioned above or of even some that may not have been mentioned. Ideally, when variables are properly controlled, curves will primarily represent the conditions imposed in the study. And so, as in Figure 3–1, we observe two similar shaped curves, with one more elevated than the other.

Examples

In another type of study, the curves for one or more groups might be different—different from each other as well as from those in Figure 3–1. Some possibilities for the shape of curves are as follows. Two groups of subjects may begin a study at the same level of achievement, but different achievement rates may occur during practice:

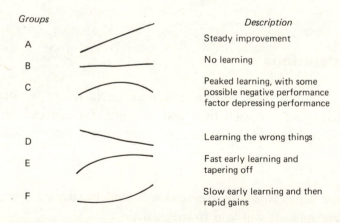

The above illustrations represent performances over trials, with better performances indicated by an elevation in the curve: The following framework is one you should use in plotting data.

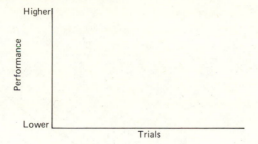

In an experiment in which two or more groups are compared in learning as a function of their respective learning conditions, we would be interested in "what works and what isn't working." The concerns are the same in an instructional program.

To re-emphasize, real performance results will not look like these curves. They may approximate them. Figures 3–2 and 3–5 indicate what "real" data might look like when illustrated. The curves assume different forms. In an experiment, a researcher might administer 15 trials to a group of subjects, who will attempt to learn a new motor task. Time on target is calculated following each trial, but in these cases only the scores of trials 1–2, 5–6, 9–10, and 14–15 are plotted.

Figure 3–2 approximates a *linear curve:* a direct relationship between practice trials and performance level. Figure 3–3 illustrates a *positively accelerated curve,* in that learning appears to be slow as first, with great improvements in the latter trials. A *negatively accelerated curve,* the reverse trend, is indicated in Figure 3–4. An S-shaped curve is illustrated in Figure 3–5, with a rapid gain at first, stability in performance in the middle, and rapid gains again toward the end.

Plateaus

Can we practice and reach a point of no more learning, even though there is still much to be learned? Perhaps you have experienced a sports situation where your learning progress was great a first, and you thought to yourself, "Nothing to it." Then everything seemed to go wrong. You hit a stalemate. Not only was progress lacking, it may have appeared that performance was worsening. Then, one day, everything went right. Performance gains were progressive—slow, but positive.

The *leveling off in performance, preceded and followed by performance gains,* has been termed a *plateau.* Although people swear to personal experiences

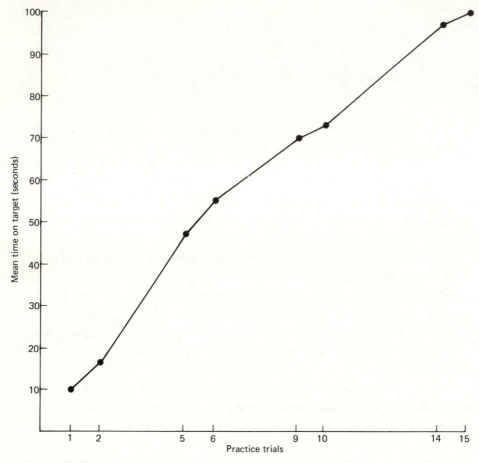

Figure 3–2. A linear curve.*

of suffering with plateaus in learning, laboratory research has not verified its existence. The very early study by Bryan and Harter in 1897 revealed a plateau for individuals attempting to acquire skill in telegraphic coding. But such evidence has been difficult to reproduce under controlled learning conditions.

Nevertheless, if plateaus do exist, they are obviously not desirable. They are frustrating. Many times learning is occurring, but we are attempting to *put together lower-order skills with more sophisticated skills.* The process may take time and patience. Other explanations are plausible, too. Consider:

(1) level of skill
(2) the demands placed on the learner

* Figures 3–2 to 3–5 from Singer, R. N., Milne, C., Magill, R., Powell, F. M., and Vachon, L. *Laboratory and Field Experiments in Motor Learning.* Springfield, Ill.: Charles C Thomas, 1975

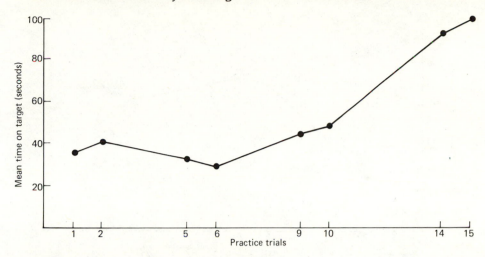

Figure 3–3. A positively accelerated curve.

(3) loss of motivation, interest, novelty
(4) fatigue
(5) lack of physical conditioning
(6) goal level too high or too low
(7) lack of understanding directions

The sensitive teacher would be on the lookout for such possible factors influencing learners. Instructional techniques must be developed to overcome these problems.

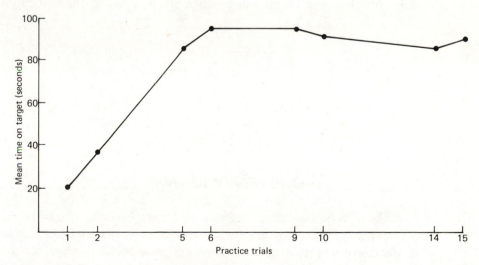

Figure 3–4. A negatively accelerated curve.

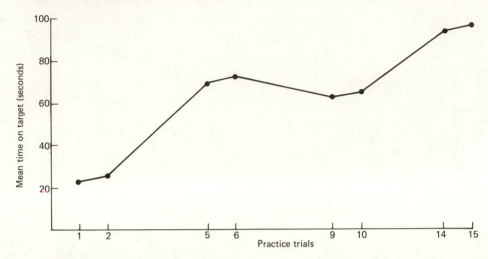

Figure 3–5. An S-shaped curve.

If you didn't want to conduct an experiment, but were interested in the progress of each student, learning curves could be plotted rather conveniently at regular intervals in some activities: swimming or running times, archery accuracy, basketball shooting, and tennis serving accuracy come to mind as examples. In other activities, subjective teacher evaluations of performance would be necessary. These are time-consuming and impose hardships on the teacher if a comprehensive evaluation is wanted. Whenever possible, individual learning curves might be kept in a class, as they are informative for both the teacher and student and possibly motivational as well.

Remember, to construct a curve, place the performance indicator and limits on the horizontal line and number of practice attempts along the vertical line:

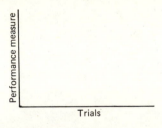

ONE NEVER KNOWS

A comic book, a pornographic magazine, or Plato's *Republic* may be far more exciting reading (at least the first two); it takes time to get used to the style of writing and format of research. I once knew a physical education major, a number of years ago, who couldn't have cared less about studying from books associated with physical education. He loved sports—it was his life. He wanted to play basketball and baseball, and did quite successfully at his college. He hoped to coach one sport or the other upon graduation. He didn't even know the meaning of research. He hated to write or read.

Then he decided to obtain a master's degree. Even a doctorate. He still wanted to coach. But not only did he learn what research and the spirit of inquiry and problem-solving was all about, he became fascinated with it. He read. He wrote. He researched. More and more. Throughout his subsequent university positions, he enjoyed a balanced life of teaching, writing, and research, and participating in a number of sports. That person was me!

I was a potential college dropout at the end of my first year in undergraduate school. Somehow, in later years, I was able to put many goals and activities together, in perspective. Reading and conducting research is one intellectually stimulating avenue to pursue. Understanding research findings and applying them to teaching and coaching situations is another avenue. I hope that you find the ideal relationship of playing to learning, and that you find it earlier in your professional career than I did.

RESEARCH

The discussion on learning curves and some other topics has already helped to introduce you to the nature of research and experimentation. Many of the statements about learning that will be made later in the book will be derived from research findings. You will need to become familiar with research protocol—how a problem worthy of study is identified, translated into an actual plan with formal procedures in order to obtain answers, and resolved or not resolved.

Perhaps you will have to undertake some readings of studies as an assignment in class. Maybe you will even be required to conduct a miniature experiment. Both kinds of assignment will give you a better feel for what research is, and make you a better consumer at the same time. Remember, in this book I am taking the liberty of interpreting and generalizing from available research. This makes it convenient for you. But don't be lazy. Read and critique original articles yourself.

THE DESIGN OF EXPERIMENTS

Experimentation is one type of research and the one used most often in the study of learning. Typically, the following steps are followed by the experimenter.
1. A *meaningful problem* is identified.

In order for a problem to be meaningful, it should have theoretical or practical significance, or both. The findings of the study might contribute to a body of knowledge, influence teaching, or both. It is considered "a problem" because we are not sure of the answer. A well-designed study would help to determine that answer.

2. A *hypothesis* is generated.

There should be some expectations in the study as to the direction of the data. These are usually based on conceptual directions, other related research findings, intuition and common sense, or all of them.

3. *Research literature* is reviewed.

An awareness of related research designs and findings and a knowledge of research and statistical techniques in general aid in the establishment of the problem and the formulation of testable hypotheses and plans for the conduct of research. The more one knows, the better ideas can be developed. Books, research articles, and the opinions of authorities contribute to understanding.

4. *Experimental procedures* are designed.

To be considered are independent and dependent variables, experimental control factors, plans to be followed, and statistics to be applied to the data.

5. The *independent variable* is the variable of interest; it is the one manipulated by the experimenter. Let's say that the experiment was to test the effectiveness of a certain instructional approach. The *independent variable* would be the use of the new approach; the *dependent variable* would be any indication of the effectiveness of this approach on the students' learning.

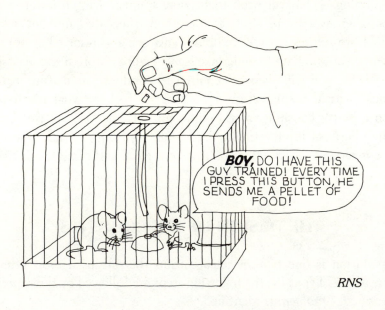

RNS

of interest. Typically, an experimental group and a control group of subjects would be formed. The experimental group would receive the special instructional approach (maybe the use of videotape) whereas the control group would not. All other conditions should remain the same for all subjects; the conditions should be *controlled* as much as possible. In some situations, it's not so easy to know who is controlling whom, as shown in the cartoon!

As to the *plan* for the investigation, we would need to determine the learning activity (task), how often and long the subjects are to be in the experiment, what learning score is to be used, and which learning measurement technique would best inform us of the relative effectiveness of the videotape apparatus in the instructional setting. Subjects are tested under controlled conditions.

6. *Statistics* are applied to data in order to make probability statements about the findings.

Are performance differences within or between groups "real"? Are they due to chance? Statistics will indicate, for instance, whether we might expect to observe the same findings as in the present study 95 per cent of the time, given the same situations repeated in the future, or 99 per cent of the time. The value percentage is determined by the researcher.

7. The *proper statistical model* is also determined by the researcher.

A *t* test would be used for a comparison of two means. Maybe we would only want to compare the final achievements of the two groups of subjects. An analysis of variance (ANOVA), or *F* test, would be used for more comparisons. It could be applied to the data if we want to determine within- and between-group differences, and any interaction. With more groups and more variables, more complex statistical models can be used. And depending on the research problem and questions raised, one or more statistical models may be more appropriate than others. A few references listed at the end of this chapter will help you to understand the nature and application of statistics.

Our design could look like this:

	Pretest	**Posttest**
Experimental group		
Control group		

If the same tests were given on two occasions, a pretest (before instruction) and a posttest (after instruction), the four cells indicate the comparisons that could be made:

a. pretest versus posttest scores, with both groups combined.
b. experimental group versus control group, with both tests combined.
c. the interaction effect between tests and groups.

In effect, we would be most interested in the third analysis. The question that would be answered is: Does one group perform any differently from the other as a function of the test? Hypothetically, we might expect the subjects to be equal at the start of the experiment (pretest) but different at the end (posttest), in favor of the experimental group. If this were true, our data might look like this:

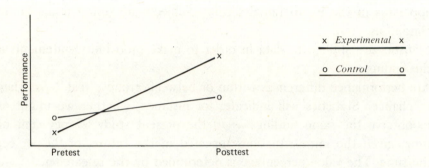

Both groups improved, but the experimental group improved more. Of course, we could have had repeated trials, maybe ten, and analyzed the data trial by trial. Other possibilities exist as well.

8. *Conclusions* are made.
Following a statistical analysis of the data, conclusions and implications are drawn. The original problem and questions are resolved, at least in this study. But these data will need to be discussed in the contest of other research findings in order to draw a more comprehensive picture of the research area.

The previous discussion should have given you a feeling for experimentation. The experiment was kept simple. It could have been made far more complex, as could the discussion on the sequential steps. As you read more and gain experience, investigations will become easier to understand. So will your ability to plan experiments.

SUMMARY

In this chapter we learned how to quantify learning. There is no direct assessment of learning, and the best indirect approach is to use some measure of performance. The more personal and situational conditions are considered and controlled for each subject or student, the more it is probable that tests will come closer in reflecting "true" learning levels.

What should constitute a learning score? Speed and accuracy measures, separately or together, are most often used in experiments to indicate improvements in learning and skill. Subjective evaluations of form, of movement skill, are made more often in the gymnasium than in the laboratory. With each of these types of measurements, there are varied techniques and approaches usually available. The nature of the learning task and the objective of the investigation will suggest what score or scores to use.

Similar problems arise with the attempt to determine the appropriate learning measure or measures. The final score, gain (improvement) score, average score, and trial-to-trial analyses of scores illustrate the most popular alternatives. Again, the purpose of the study will influence decisions.

Learning curves are graphic representations of the same data collected on the same people on two or more occasions. They reveal trends in the data. Statistical analysis is needed to affirm observed trends. Research, and especially experiments, provides the basis for the science of motor learning. In turn, this information can provide the support structure for the science of teaching and coaching.

REFERENCES AND SUGGESTED READINGS

Bruning, J. L. and Kintz, B. L. *Computational handbook of statistics.* Glenview, Ill.: Scott, Foresman and Co., 1977.

Dunham, P. Learning and performance. *Research Quarterly,* 1971, 42, 334–337.

Keppel, G. and Saufley, W. H. *Introduction to design and Analysis.* San Francisco: W. H. Freeman and Co., 1980.

Safrit, M. J., Spray, J. A., and Diewert, G. L. Methodological Issues in short-term motor memory research. *Journal of Motor Behavior,* 1980, 12, 13–28.

Singer, R. N. *Motor learning and human performance,* third edition. New York: Macmillan Publishing Co., Inc., 1980, chapter 3.

Singer, R. N., Milne, C., Magill, R., Powell, F. M., and Vachon, L. *Laboratory and field experiments in motor learning.* Springfield, Ill.: Charles C Thomas, 1975, Chapters 1 and 2.

4

MOTOR LEARNING ACTIVITIES AND TASKS

So many routine recreational and occupational activities involve movement that an incredible number of them could be viewed as motor activities. We, in this book, are concerned with the most obvious: large muscle or gross motor learning tasks. Athletic, physical education, dance, and recreational activities demand the effective integration of many muscle groups of the body. Skill is determined by the appropriate sequence and timing of movements in space to achieve an objective.

The body of information about motor learning and behavior has come largely from efforts in research laboratories. Typically, different types of skills are examined in the laboratory from those scrutinized in the world of the physical educator. Both sources of information are valuable. But, as we emphasized in Chapter 1, the laboratory affords the opportunity to control many more factors than is the case in real-world learning situations.

Our discussion will begin with an analysis of the motor learning tasks usually used in the research. Classification systems of motor activities have been formulated by scholars, and these will be presented. Commonalities among tasks and distinctions among groups of them, once identified, lead to a better understanding of what special instructional factors need to be considered.

55

REAL-WORLD ACTIVITIES

Virtually all of the sports activities have been analyzed both as to a comparison of the effectiveness of alternative learning approaches on achievement in the activity in general, and as to a comparison of different techniques as used with the particular sports skill. Furthermore, the relationship of certain psychological factors to skill in a particular sport has been investigated on occasion.

In the second case, scores on laboratory tests measuring such parameters as reaction time, limb movement speed, balance, coordination, kinesthesis, and depth perception have been correlated with achievement in specific sports. Sometimes, athletes representing different sports have been compared for these attributes. These, of course, are not experimental studies but rather descriptive studies. They indicate the "going-togetherness" of selected factors, factors that might contribute to learning and achievement.

The *Research Quarterly Index,* issues of 1964 (for 1930–1960) and 1979 (for 1930–1976) as well as in each December issue, provides author and subject indexes for the articles in that journal. Likewise, *Completed Research in Health, Physical Education, and Recreation,* published annually since 1959, is a very valuable source. Titles and abstracts for theses and dissertations finished each year in the United States, and titles for research on motor skills in many journals, are presented in this publication. Consequently, if you are interested in research on various physical education activities, these are good sources. Indexed are all types of investigations on motor behavior, sport, fitness, and the like. You will have to locate the sport and psychological attributes of your choice.

The same is true in the first case given in the first paragraph in this section. Experimental studies comparing methods and techniques may be found in the sources just mentioned for many real-world activities. You may be interested only in sport. But studies in other literature may be retrieved that deal with the learning of typing, musical skills, vocational skills, speech and other matter.

Techniques and practice conditions to improve learning and retention in real-world activities were investigated by psychologists as early as 1905. Edgar Swift used a sort of juggling task in studies reported in 1905 and 1910, and a typing task in 1906. He demonstrated that skill in these activities is retained over long periods of no practice. Karl Lashley investigated the acquisition of skill in archery in 1915, with five groups of subjects. Results indicated a greater proficiency for the groups that shot less each day and had their practice periods distributed over a long period. For instance, the group that shot twelve arrows a day improved 47 per cent whereas the sixty-shot group showed an improvement of 27 per cent. Herbert Murphy studied practice conditions for acquiring skill in javelin throwing in 1916. All groups received 34 practice sessions. However, practicing three times or once a week was favored over five times a week. These early studies provide a historical behavioral perspective of research on skills, specifically on the acquisition and retention of skill. Countless procedures and conditions have been investigated with many different tasks since those years.

What has it all led to? With regard to research directly on teaching, or with implications for teaching, interpretations vary as to its value. Lawrence Locke, writing in a 1977 issue of *Quest,* is critical about research on teaching physical education. He considers its nature, direction, and practical utility to be in a dismal state. Cautiously optimistic, nevertheless, he writes that "the new science of research on teaching physical education is only a fledgling, but if its significance is recognized it can be nurtured and made to grow" (p. 13). Yet M. Dunkin and B. Biddle in their book, *The Study of Teaching* (1974), state that sufficient research has been completed concerning teaching (in general). They believe that "the study of teaching is the heartland of the research effort that should govern education" (p. viii).

Perhaps after you finish reading this book you will be in a better position to determine for yourself the value of research in motor learning for instructional and self-teaching situations.

LABORATORY TASKS AND TESTS

One of the major purposes of those scholars who undertake research in the laboratory is to assess and observe behavior as accurately as possible. Refined instrumentation yielding quantitative and sensitive data helps to achieve this objective. Special apparatuses may be used to assess the status, level, or degree of presence of some personal characteristic (sometimes termed *ability* or *trait*). The other and primary purpose of apparatuses is to present learning tasks. In both cases, equipment has been purchased or constructed, or some combination may be created.

Personal Characteristics

One of the more challenging goals is to find a task to measure a particular personal characteristic, like an aptitude, ability, or trait. Presumably, these terms represent enduring characteristics of people; they are somewhat stable throughout life. Some scholars disagree with this notion. They feel that such capabilities can be modified through learning.

In principle, the degree of development of abilities related to achievement in a task or sport should aid in the learning and performance of it. Certain abilities underlie success in related activities.

For example, to perform well in baseball probably requires spatial-orientation ability (awareness of objects in space surrounding the situation, e.g., the ball hit to the fielder or pitched to the batter); response integration (to coordinate eye, hand, trunk, and leg movements for purposeful behavior); the ability to endure and tolerate many hours of practice; and the like. The same is true in all ball sports, like tennis, volleyball, soccer, and racketball.

There are many abilities and even more skills representing these abilities. But even a single ability, like the one labelled *balance*, may assume many forms. The ability to balance can be demonstrated in such skills as standing on one foot without falling, walking a narrow rail without losing equilibrium, maintaining a straddled pivoted board in a horizontal position, landing on the trampoline in an upright position, spiking a volleyball without losing composure, and shooting a jump shot in basketball while landing correctly. Different types of balance contribute to success in each of these activities.

In most, if not all, skills no one ability underlies achievement. Rather, the interaction of a number of abilities, along with proper extensive task-specific practice, contributes to achievement in an activity. Therefore, the usefulness of ability tests to predict achievement in particular tasks depends on the relationship between the ability task and the criterion (learning) task.

Apparatuses to Assess Personal Characteristics

(1) Reaction Time

In the middle of the eighteenth century, a piece of equipment to test reaction time was invented. It was the first apparatus used for psychological experimentation, and although it has been refined through the ages, the basic design remains the same.

Experimentally speaking, *reaction time refers to the time elapsed between the presentation of a stimulus and the initiation of a response.*

Typically in everyday situations we interpret reaction time in a more general way. We might observe a baseball batter's response to the pitched ball and casually comment on the quickness of his or her batting reactions. The same holds true with the hockey or soccer goalie. Usually, though, we are not only observing the athlete's reactions but his or her movement responses as well. That is to say, we not only witness the stimulus (an environmental event) and time lag before the response but the nature of the response itself. Since the entire movement occurs so quickly in typical situations, a pure indication of reaction time is extremely hard to ascertain under such realistic circumstances as athletic events.

Thus, the laboratory setting becomes a means of more accurately measuring reaction time. In the simplest reaction time equipment, the subject presses a finger on a button or key and releases it with the presentation of some stimulus, which is usually auditory or visual in nature. Time elapsed is recorded on a chronoscope (timer) and thus a measure of reaction is obtained.

Figure 4–1 contains an illustration of a simple reaction time apparatus. With this equipment, the object is for the subject to press the key down rather than releasing it. A timing mechanism is connected to the reaction time unit, and a timer is presented in Figure 4–2. The digital clock constructed by the Marietta Company measures to 1/100, although other companies have built timers that record time intervals of up to 1/1000 second.

In most real-life situations, an individual is faced with a number of stimuli and responses among which he or she must discriminate to respond correctly. It is rare when, as in a laboratory, a person is told the correct stimulus and

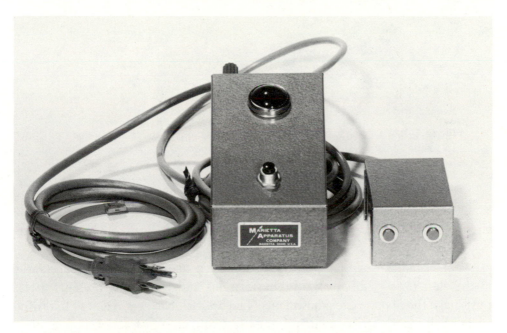

Figure 4–1. Simple reaction time apparatus. The subject is instructed to hold the response key down. The experimenter then pushes one of two buttons on his control box which will deliver a light or auditory stimulus and will start a timer. The subject is to release pressure on the key as response to the stimulus, at which time the timer stops. (From Marietta Apparatus Company, 118 Maple Street, Marietta, Ohio.)

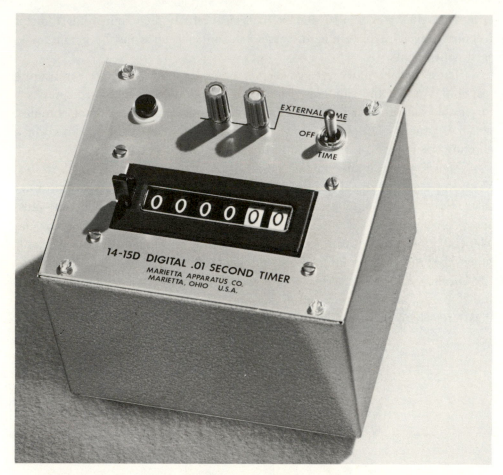

Figure 4–2A. Digital 1/100th-second stopclock. (From Marietta Apparatus Company, 118 Maple Street, Marietta, Ohio.)

where it will occur beforehand, thereby being able to wait patiently for the occurrence.

For instance, when an individual drives a car he or she must be constantly on the alert for a number of possible situations and, when one presents itself, must make the appropriate adjustments. The baseball batter is required to distinguish a ball from a strike, a curve from a fast ball, all in a fraction of a second.

The ability to respond correctly (quickly and accurately) to one of a number of possible choices can be measured in the laboratory with a choice of discrimination reaction-time apparatus. The one pictured in Figure 4–3 contains three stimulus lights and three response keys. The investigator can preset the key that is to be correctly associated with a given stimulus. The instrument measures

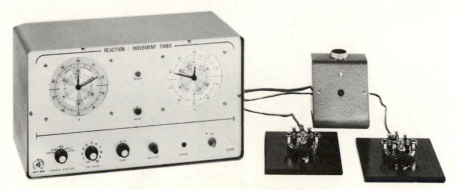

Figure 4–2B. The reaction/movement timer. This two-clock reaction timer has been designed specifically to discriminate between both reaction time and movement time. This is accomplished by means of two response keys and two clocks which are started simultaneously. The first clock is deactivated when the subject removes his or her hand from the depressed key, while the second clock is not deactivated until the second key is depressed. In this way, it is possible to obtain a measure of reaction time to the first key, total reaction time to the second key, and movement time from the first key to the second key. (From Lafayette Instrument Co., Lafayette, Indiana.)

perception (ability to identify the desired response to a particular stimulus) as well as speed of reaction of movement.

(2) Kinesthesis

Visual and movement senses play an important role in motor performance. *The awareness of the body in space and the relationship of its parts, the sensation of movement, refers to kinesthesis,* also known as *proprioception.* The outstanding athlete usually "feels" the movement performed. He or she must be in control of the body, be aware of positioning and accuracy of body and limbs, and perform with efficiency and effectiveness.

The beginning golfer is often told to be concerned more with the swing and how it feels than with where the ball goes. Presumably, concentration on correct sequences of appropriate responses will eventually lead to desired outcomes, with the need to be conscious of the swing having been overcome. Certainly a gymnast needs to sense the relationship of body parts during the execution of a skill. In every activity, kinesthesis underlies achievement.

The physical education research field contains many tests, both laboratory and nonlaboratory oriented, to measure this sense. One example of a kinesthetic task, or specifically a positioning task, is pictured in Figure 4–4. The subject moves an arm and points to a predesignated point on the board, which is laid out in degrees up to 180. He or she is then blindfolded and attempts to replicate the movement. Since the board is laid out in degrees, it is possible to determine quantitatively the number of degrees the subject is off the target point.

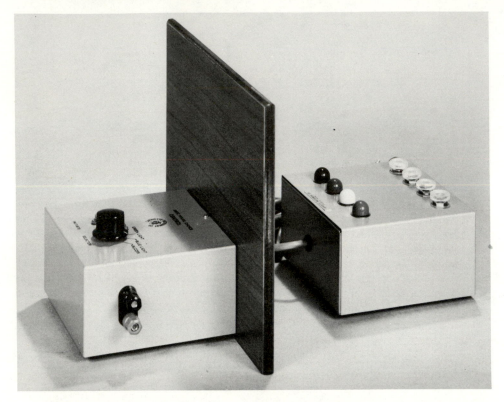

Figure 4–3. Visual choice reaction time apparatus. The apparatus consists of two units—an experimenter's control module and a subject's stimulus-display-response module. These modules are isolated by a 15-foot cable to eliminate the chance of any spurious stimulus cues. The subject module includes four lights, a buzzer, and four response keys. The experimenter selects which stimulus light goes on, and the timer runs until the correct response key is depressed. When the correct response is made, the stimulus light goes off and the timer is stopped. (From Lafayette Instrument Company, P.O. Box 1279, Lafayette, Indiana.)

There is no general *kinesthetic sense.* It is *specific* to the test and the part of the body involved in the skill. Kinesthesis is apparently related to successful motor performance, and like balance, coordination, and other abilities, must be developed specifically for a particular task.

(3) Sense Sensitivity

The ability to notice small differences in stimulation is an important attribute. Naturally, the further apart levels of stimulation are for a given stimulus, the easier detection becomes. The perceiving of just-noticeable differences, or sensitivity, in sensations is associated with an area of study called *psychophysics.*

Wrestlers must demonstrate sensitivity to the changes in touch and pressure they feel from the opponent's tactics in order to block escapes or escape themselves from changing offensive maneuvers. Quick reactions to the slightest pressure help to determine control in a match.

A traditional method of measuring sense sensitivity involves the use of weighted cylinders (see Figure 4–5). These weights are graduated in 50-gram steps from 100 to 600 grams. Typically, the subject is required to lift a standard weight, then a comparison weight, and decide whether the comparison weight is heavier or lighter than the standard weight. Obviously, the further removed the two weights are from each other, the more easily differences and the correct direction of the differences are detected.

(4) Balance

The ability to maintain one's posture throughout the execution of various movements is another attribute underlying success in sports. The skilled athlete does not fall on his or her face during performance but instead demonstrates body composure and equilibrium. There are many, many occasions when an individual is required to show skill in balancing himself or herself beyond merely standing still and erect. There exist many tests to measure balancing skill as well.

We might consider two types of balance—*static* and *dynamic. Static balance*

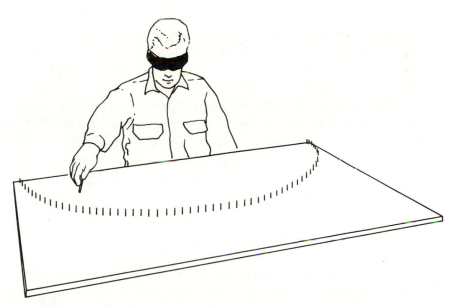

Figure 4–4. Positioning test. The blindfolded subject attempts to replicate a previous point at a peg.

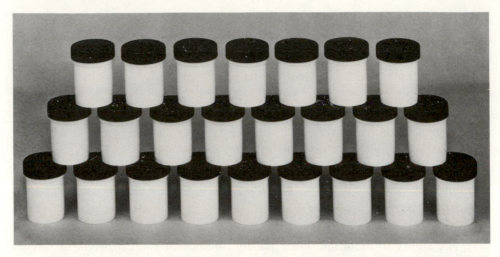

Figure 4–5. Weighed Cylinders. This set of weights consists of two series composing a total of 24 weights. The light series ranges from 75 to 125 grams in 5 gram intervals with two weights each weighing 100 grams. The heavy series ranges from 175 to 225 grams in 5 gram intervals with two weights each weighing 200 grams. The weights can be used to demonstrate many psychophysical and perceptual phenomena. (From Lafayette Instrument Co., Lafayette, Indiana.)

can be evaluated by a person's ability to stand perfectly still, with any minimal body movement being recorded on an *ataxiagraph*. Or balance can be measured through tests in which the subject must execute a *series of controlled movements on a stationary base*. Walking on a rail or a long piece of narrow wood is a good example of a static base on which a person demonstrates dynamic activity in order to remain in balance. Therefore, we have a combination of static and dynamic balance. Hopping from one object to another while attempting to maintain balance is another example.

Examples in sport where stable balance is demanded are easy to find. The basketball player dribbles the ball quickly, changes direction, stops short, shoots a jump shot, and lands on his or her feet. Throughout the entire sequence of fast action, the player is demonstrating skills in moving and controlling the body in the way he or she wants. The football quarterback receives the ball from the center, pedals back quickly, dodges one onrushing lineman, another one, runs to one side, then the other, and throws the ball just as he is hit by an opposing team member. He does not hit the turf until another force causes him to do so.

A different form of balance is registered by the water skier and trampolinist. These athletes demonstrate the ability to balance *dynamically*, or, in other words, *to execute movements on an unstable platform or base*. Thus they are moving and attempting to perform skills on yielding surfaces.

In the laboratory, an apparatus used to measure this type of balance is a stabilometer. There are a number of differently constructed stabilometers, but they all work on the same basic principle. The subject straddles the moveable platform and attempts to keep it stationary. Throughout a designated period of time, say, 30 seconds, he or she attempts to maintain the platform in a desired position, and time is recorded on a *chronoscope*. One type of stabilometer is illustrated in Figure 4–6.

(5) Mechanical Ability (Eye-hand Precision)

Underlying success in executing many industrial tasks is the capacity to perform fine eye-hand manipulative, precise tasks. Dexterity with the fingers is needed by the pianist also. Most sports demand more gross body movements than the type of tasks we typically think of as representing mechanical ability; nevertheless, in many ball sports precision eye-hand coordination is a factor.

Most tests of mechanical ability require precision and speed of movement on the part of the subject. The Purdue Pegboard Test, illustrated in Figure 4–7A, is a widely distributed test. There are a number of tasks one could perform on this test, the simplest of which is to have the subject place the pegs in the holes as fast as possible. The Pennsylvania Bi-Manual Worksample, Figure 4–7B, is another frequently employed hand dexterity test, requiring the placement of small irregular objects into appropriate places. The responses must be accurate and the time elapsed to complete the test is recorded.

(6) Coordination

One of the most often used terms, and yet it is very difficult to define accurately, is the word *coordination*. We talk in terms of someone being coordinated, someone else not; a coordinated effort; a coordinated swing; and a coordinated performance. But what do we really mean? How do we measure a person's coordination?

It is probably best to think of coordination as referring to performance in a specific task, in terms of objectives accomplished through movement patterns with efficient and effective use of the musculature. More complex tasks require more coordination. The type of coordination needed for a successful golf swing is obviously different from that involved in playing a piano or serving a tennis ball.

Almost any motor test can be a test of a person's coordination, among other things. Sports skills represent coordinated movement patterns; that is, movements are *spatially* and *temporally* organized. Parts of the body involved in the execution of an act move into appropriate places at the right time in proper sequence. In the laboratory, two of the more common coordination tasks

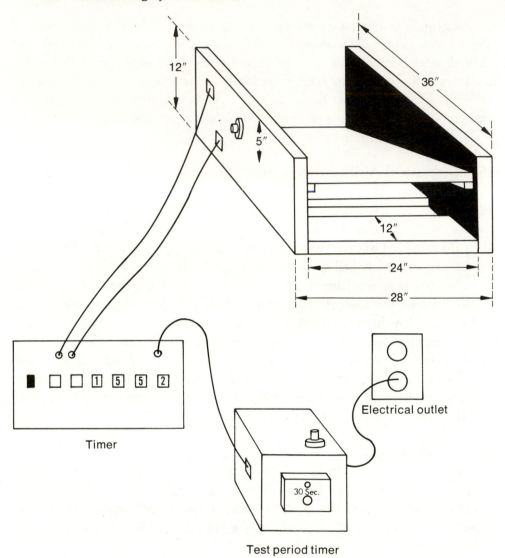

Figure 4–6. Stabilometer. The apparatus consists of a tilting platform approximately 24″ wide × 36″ long pivoted in the center with micro-switches installed to sense when the platform is in balanced position during the test cycle. The controls consist of a timer to set the duration of the test period and a clock to accumulate the total "on balance" time.

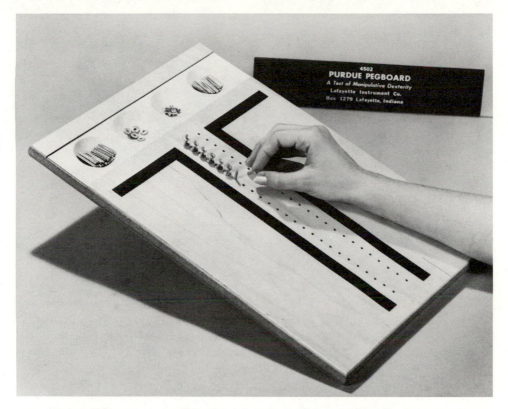

Figure 4–7a. Purdue pegboard test. In order to measure manual dexterity, pegs, collars, and washers are assembled. (From Lafayette Instrument Company, P.O. Box 1279, Lafayette, Indiana.)

use the pursuit rotor and star-tracing (stabilimeter) apparatuses, and these will be discussed in context of the next section.

Apparatuses Used in Learning Situations

The researcher interested in the psychological aspects of behavior is concerned not only with measuring characteristics but with determining the effects of environmental manipulation on the learning process as well. There are many variables that might have a bearing on the effectiveness with which we learn anything. The teacher relies on the results of studies dealing with these variables to provide direction in the selection of a teaching approach.

Although factors that might influence learning can be altered and tested for effects in the classroom situation, it is probably easier to control more possible

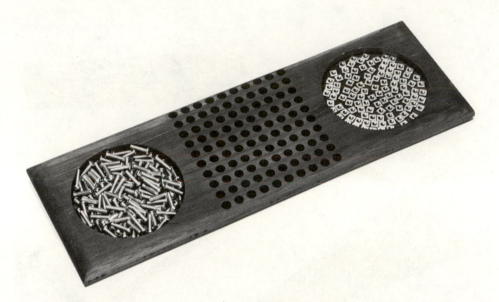

Figure 4–7b. Pennsylvania Bi-Manual Worksample. This task combines the basic elements of a relatively simple work situation. The examinee, seated before the 8″ × 24″ board, grasps a nut between thumb and index finger of left hand, and a bolt with thumb and index finger of right hand; turns the bolt into the nut, and places in holes in the board. There are 100 nut-and-bolt combinations. Twenty of these are for practice work and 80 are to be done under timing. Thus, the test combines: finger dexterity of both hands, whole movement of both arms, eye-hand coordination, bimanual coordination, and ability to use both hands in cooperation. (From American Guidance Service, Inc., Circle Pines, Minnesota.)

interacting variables in the laboratory. The researcher selects an apparatus that fulfills personal objectives for the particular experiment. Many of those pieces of equipment already mentioned could be incorporated into a study of learning. It is most important that whatever learning apparatus is decided upon yield highly accurate results.

A little later in this section of the book, we will discuss various factors that have been manipulated by investigators in their attempt to gain a clearer understanding of the learning process. Reward versus punishment, continual versus spaced practice, transfer effects from one learned task to another to be learned, and many more potential influences on the learning of a skill are to be considered. Two apparatuses frequently used in these types of investigation are the *pursuit rotor* and the *stabilimeter*. Following a description of them, a brief example of an experiment employing either piece of equipment will be presented.

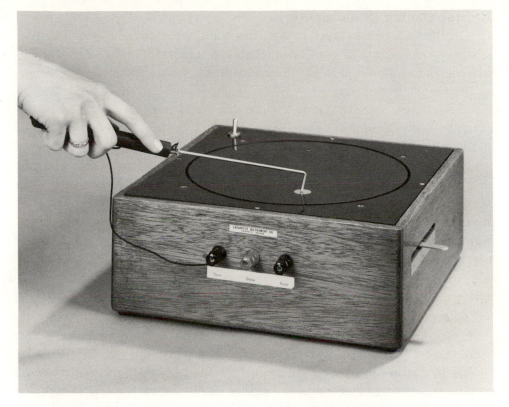

Figure 4–8. The pursuit rotor apparatus. (From Lafayette Instrument Company, P.O. Box 1279, Lafayette, Indiana.)

(1) Pursuit Rotor

In experimental studies where researchers are investigating the learning of motor skills, the pursuit rotor is the apparatus most found in the published research. The apparatus is relatively simple, although some of the more elaborate pursuit rotors are fairly expensive.

The pursuit rotor consists of a turntable that typically revolves at a designated speed, usually 60 rpm, with a small disc on it. The subject holds a stylus probe in one hand and attempts to maintain contact with the disc as the turntable moves. Time in contact is recorded for each practice session, which usually lasts 20 seconds or so. This type of activity is called a *tracking task*, for the subject continually attempts to "track down" the moving disc and maintain contact with it. A pursuit rotor is illustrated in Figure 4–8.

(2) Star-tracing (Stabilimeter)

In this task, the subject attempts to trace the pattern of a star. The goal is to move as quickly as possible through the pattern, without touching the side boundaries of the path, as these constitute errors. Therefore, speed and accuracy are both important.

Sometimes, to make the task more difficult, a mirror is attached to the apparatus, with the subject's direct view of the star pattern blocked by a shield. In this case, one must look into the mirror and perform the task, which now becomes a reversed task as he or she needs to go in the opposite direction from what appears in the mirror. If it is an electrically wired apparatus, the star pattern is grooved, and if the stylus which the subject is using touches the side at any time, an error is recorded on a counter. These errors are cumulatively added and time is recorded for each trial. One such piece of equipment may be seen in Figure 4–9. A person's score constitutes the number of errors plus time recorded (the less the better of both) in conjunction with distance traversed.

A representative investigation in which the pursuit rotor, stabilimeter, or some other equipment might be useful to study learning phenomena is the following. Suppose we wanted to determine which is more effective: to learn the task by continually practicing it through twenty trials with minimal or almost no rest pauses, to wait one minute between each trial, or possibly to rest five

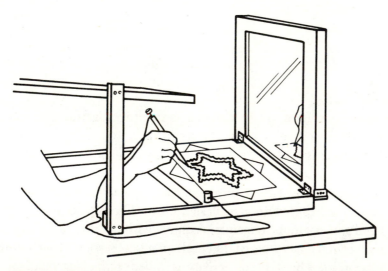

Figure 4–9. Star-tracing task. The star is traced as accurately as possible with the subject viewing it in the mirror. (*From Fulton, R. Speed and accuracy in learning movements.* Archives of Psychology, *1945, 300.*)

minutes between every trial. Physical educators and coaches teach skills and are faced with the problem of having the students either practice a skill repeatedly or rest after a certain number of trials. Or they might practice other skills interchangeably instead of resting. If foul shooting is to be perfected, should 50 consecutive attempts be made at the basket or should they be shot in groups of ten with five-minute rest pauses after each ten attempts?

Returning to the experimental study, three groups of subjects might be formed. One group would practice for 20 consecutive trials on the apparatus; a second group would rest one minute in between trials; and a third group would pause five minutes. Performances on the last trial would be compared between the groups to determine the most effective practice method. The good feature of a laboratory study of these practice effects is that most if not all subjects come to the situation without prior experience on that task. (In basketball foul shooting, this would certainly not be the case.) Practice effects and trends can more readily be seen and less influenced by other variables in the laboratory learning task.

(3) Computer-managed Tasks

The pursuit rotor and stabilimeter are very simple pieces of equipment, and offer unique learning experiences to subjects, without much cost to the experimenter or knowledge of operation needed. Many other tasks like these can be purchased or constructed.

It is also possible to use computers to manage learning tasks. Once the subject's task is constructed, it can be hooked up to a computer. Operations are guided by programs. The experimenter can be completely out of the picture. The computer can display instructions, regulate the learning apparatus, record the data, store them, and even analyze them. An experimenter control system is depicted in Figure 4–10, as is the SMA (Serial Manipulation Apparatus), a learning task that requires the subject to quickly manipulate the appropriate object on the panel in response to a cue. The relative effectiveness of certain *learner strategies* in skill acquisition and retention can be examined with this test. (For a full discussion of the nature of learner strategies, see Chapter 9, *The Highly Skilled.*)

We have just reviewed representative pieces of equipment that can be involved in motor learning experiments. Considering all the rest, and the tremendous number of real-world motor activities and tasks, it is of interest and practical concern to determine if some means can be used to determine things in common about them. Approaches to the classification of motor tasks will now be discussed, as well the potential value of these attempts.

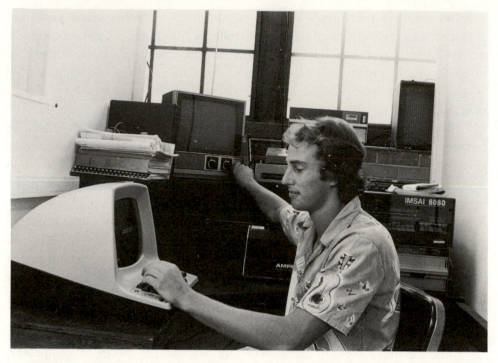

Figure 4–10A. The experimenter in a computer-managed learning task situation.

TASK CLASSIFICATION SYSTEMS

Theories are formulated in an attempt to organize many research findings, to provide unity and make sense out of many research thrusts. Task classifications serve a similar purpose. A higher-order task classification system is a *taxonomy*. It is a means of classifying objects or phenomena in such a way that useful relationships among them are established. A hierarchical progression of behaviors is included. The psychomotor domain of behavior has resisted a meaningful taxonomic structure. However, there are different approaches to classifying activities, to determine what things have in common and how they differ. The reason for determining pertinent task characteristics that will allow us to "clump" tasks into distinct groups is that

(1) learning theory can be developed more systematically (with special consideration for types of tasks);

(2) teachers and curriculum builders are helped in their effort to plan learning experiences and evaluation measures for specific objectives.

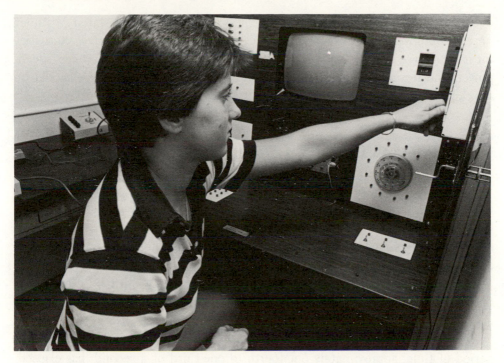

Figure 4–10B. The subject learning a computer-managed task involving the Serial Manipulation Apparatus.

Let us proceed from the cruder and more obvious classification distinctions to those that are more interesting and potentially valuable for the teacher. The primary purpose of a classification system is to avoid having to consider every activity as a separate entity requiring unique considerations. When activities possess properties in common, this means that similar teaching approaches can be effective across them.

Degree of Bodily Involvement

Along a continuum, activities can be classified as being primarily *gross motor skills* or *fine motor skills.* Gross motor skills involve large muscles of the body. Precision movements (eye-hand) are usually associated with fine motor skills. The classification of activities as being primarily gross or fine does not serve any special function except that there may be special considerations for (1) different learning procedures and processes, and (2) levels and types of fitness unique to each category.

We must always remember what appears to be obvious: practice must be of high quality and duration if improvement is going to be demonstated. Without *fitness* appropriate for the task, practice will not be too effective. Activities must be analyzed carefully for physical demands, and strength, endurance, speed, power, and flexibility associated with the particular learning activity should be developed within each student.

Length and Control of Movement

Skills can be classified in at least three ways with regard to length and control of movement. Here we will consider discrete, serial, and continuous tasks. Discrete tasks have well defined beginnings and endings, and usually they are very brief in nature. Pushing a switch, throwing a ball, or pressing a key are tasks that are discrete in nature.

Sometimes tasks are performed so quickly that they must be preplanned, or preprogrammed. They are *ballistic* in nature. The control over the movement is, in a sense, *feedforward*, and is considered *open-loop* as a system. In an open-loop task, once the movement is initiated; it cannot be modified until a certain period of time, approximately one-fourth to one-third of a second, has elapsed. By this time, many kinds of movements can be completed. Knowing this, perhaps you will not realize why the best hitters in baseball, like Hank Aaron and Rod Carew, developed a tremendous ability not to commit while batting until the last possible moment. The decision, to swing or not to swing, cannot be reversed in time to make a meaningful difference.

Chewing gum is a continuous process, another type of activity that is essentially preplanned and open-loop in nature. Once begun, we don't need to think about chewing. It's done as if automatically. However, many *continuous tasks* do require conscious attention, and depend on *feedback* for on-going control, regulation, and correction of movements. A system is considered *closed-loop* when it operates this way.

Serial tasks are continuous but require a set series of operations or sequence of events. You open the car door with a key, put it in the ignition, turn it while placing your foot on the gas, take your foot off the pedal, put the transmission in "Drive" or "Reverse," depending on the situation, and apply your foot to the gas pedal again while controlling the steering wheel with your hands. This sequence of operations, acts done in a *serial* manner, is typical. However, once driving on the highway, the act becomes *continuous*. Depending on signs, lights, traffic flow, pedestrians, road disturbances, and other factors, driving occurs under preplanned and feedback conditions. Switching in control, from deliberate conscious intervention to a sense of automaticity, happens in many sports as well as in driving a car. In activities that are slow enough, there is time to operate under closed-loop, or feedback, control if needed. Best performers seem to know how and when to *switch* from open-loop to closed-loop control and vice versa, assuming the activity is of such a nature as to allow for switching.

Environmental Control

In E. C. Poulton's (1957) classic work, tasks were classified as to situational demands on the learner/performer. He categorized tasks as *open* or *closed*. In a closed skill, the environment is stable and there is no concern for rapid perceptual adjustments to changing and possibly unpredictable events. It is *self-paced*. Examples are bowling, golf, the foul shot in basketball, and the serve in tennis.

Open skills require the performer to anticipate and to make decisions about response adaptation in a brief period of time. They are *externally-paced*, in that the situation paces the person. In wrestling, soccer, or a football game, although plans may have been established, there must be a sense of adaptability to potentially altered or unplanned occurrences.

Many open skills may first be learned under more controlled and stable conditions. But then they need to be practiced under a variety of conditions. Closed skills are practiced more mechanically, to achieve habit-like properties. Thus, the strategies for achieving in open skills and in closed skills will be somewhat different.

Cognitive Involvement

A few investigators have separated cognitive-perceptual and motor components of tasks. Obviously, activities involve the learning of many strategies and tactics. Some activities are rather repetitive in terms of movements involved. Figure 4–11 illustrates extreme examples of activities with different levels of mental involvement in them. The effectiveness with which a person handles an information load will depend on the learning of pertinent strategies that facilitate cue identification, anticipation, decision-making, and movement program selection.

Feedback Availability

In almost every activity, *feedback* is available to a person as a result of his or her own actions. It may be *ongoing*, during the activity, if the activity is of long enough duration. If the movements are slow enough, adjustments

Low cognitive   High cognitive

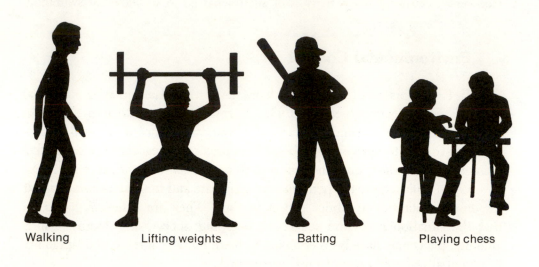

Walking   Lifting weights   Batting   Playing chess

High motor   Low motor

Figure 4–11. Relationships of cognitive to motor demands in different activities.

can be made. Or, it may be *terminal*. That is, we may see or feel how an act was just performed, or what the outcome of the act was.

Skilled performance is often evidenced by a learner's ability to use response-produced feedback. A highly skilled performer knows which feedback cues are relevant and when they should be attended to, while the less skilled person may unnecessarily consider extraneous and irrelevant cues. From the teacher's point of view, then, it pays to recognize which activities offer sufficient feedback to learners and which do not. When feedback is available, the student must learn when and how to use it. When it is unavailable or available in a limited way, additional assistance by the teacher will be required.

OVERVIEW OF TASK CLASSIFICATION

As we have seen, categories of motor tasks can be identified on the basis of commonalities with regard to situational demands, types of control a person can exert, and types of behavior required. Classifications can consider any one or combination of factors, such as

(1) bodily involvement.
(2) duration of movement.
(3) pacing conditions.
(4) cognitive involvement.
(5) feedback availability.

Basically, the objective of this material is to stress the importance of *task* or *activity analysis. An analysis of the demands placed on the learner of each activity* (and these *demands change* as skill increases), *is of paramount importance.* Instructional plans must incorporate ideas that will help learners to meet these challenges. Singer and Dick (1980) have suggested a systems approach to teaching in physical education, and one facet has to do with task analysis and the sequencing of instruction.

On the other hand, *person analysis* is very valuable, too. Recognition of individual capabilities, skill level, motivation, emotions, and other factors leads to more sensitive individualized instruction.

TASK ANALYSIS

Analysis of task demands and the relative complexity of the major considerations in the learning/performance of the task can be carried further than has been discussed so far. John Billing (1980) has recently attempted to identify the major factors that contribute to task difficulty (see Figure 4–12). Four major categories involved in the motor act are:

perception,
decision-making,
the nature of the act itself,
and feedback availability.

Within each of these categories, items are found that can contribute to the complexity of each of them, and in turn, to the entire act itself.

The purpose behind this effort is to offer the teacher or student a greater understanding of and appreciation for task complexity. But merely to say an activity is difficult is not enough. By specifying what specifically may contribute to difficulties a student will have in learning an activity, a more systematic and meaningful plan for instruction can be devised.

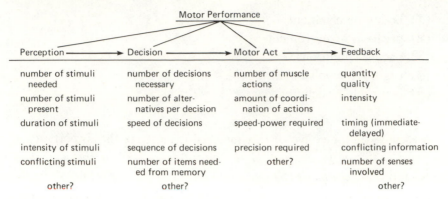

Figure 4–12. Motor acts analyzed according to the complexity of each subcomponent. (From Billing, J. An overview of task complexity. *Motor Skills: Theory Into Practice.* 1980, 4, 18–23.)

Billing (1980) offers a practical application of his task analysis model for instruction in tennis. He suggests the following:

> An analysis of the tennis forehand might help to exemplify how each component contributes to the total complexity of the task and to serve as an example of how complexity can be reduced to produce a learning progression. In the context of a tennis game, hitting an effective forehand would require perception of the court, net height, trajectory of the incoming ball, speed of the ball, opponent's position, etc. Reduction of the perceptual complexity could include: beginning the stroke from a specific court position, having the ball delivered from a standard position, delivering the ball with a consistent trajectory, reducing the speed of the ball, using colored balls and a contrasting background, and having no spin on the ball which would cause an unexpected bounce. The decisions as to what stroke, where placed, how hard, when to hit and what to do after the stroke can all be predetermined and specified to the learners to reduce their decisions making complexity. The difficulty of the motor actions themselves could be reduced by beginning from a side-to-net position, starting with the racket back and weight on the rear foot before the ball is delivered, swinging with moderate speed, and not requiring that the ball be hit into the court. Complexity in interpreting feedback could be reduced by provision for descriptive information after each trial, identifying specific corrections to be made, reinforcing and correcting with significant intensity, providing for both concurrent and terminal feedback after each trial, and stressing awareness of the kinesthetic sensations when performing the skill as well as providing verbal and visual feedback if possible.

> Similarly the complexity of any motor performance may be systematically increased by adjusting the complexity of any component. This systematic increasing of complexity provides an obvious format for constructing appropriate learning progressions (pp. 22–23).

SUMMARY

In this chapter, the goals were two-fold. One goal was to inform you of real-world and laboratory activities that have been used in motor learning investigations. The emphasis was on the laboratory setting, as much more published research in motor learning has occurred in the laboratory than in classrooms or gymnasiums. Tighter experimental controls are possible in the laboratory.

The second goal was to indicate directions in motor task classification systems. Classification systems help us to group activities in terms of elements in common, with each category nonetheless differing from other groups of activities in certain characteristics. The real value should be realized by the teacher, who has responsibility for the management of instruction. Further, appreciation of the teacher for task demands, learner control processes, and desirable performance behaviors should lead to more effective teaching and more rapid learning.

REFERENCES AND SUGGESTED READINGS

Billing, J. An overview of task complexity. *Motor Skills: Theory Into Practice,* 1980, 4, 18–23.

Cromwell, C., Weibell, F. J., Pfeiffer, E. A., and Usselman, L. B. *Biomedical instrumentation and measurements.* Englewood Cliffs, N.J.: Prentice-Hall, 1973.

Farrell, J. E. The classification of physical education skills. *Quest,* 1975, 14, 63–68.

Fleishman, E. A. Toward a taxonomy of human performance. *American Psychologist,* 1975, 30, 1127–1149.

Gentile, A. M., Higgins, J. R., Miller, E. A., and Rosen, B. M. The structure of motor tasks. *Mouvement,* 1975, 7, 11–28.

Harrow, A. J. *A taxonomy of the psychomotor domain.* New York: David McKay, 1971.

Kriefeldt, G. A dynamic model of behavior in a discrete open-loop self-paced motor skill. *IEEE Transactions on Systems, Man, and Cybernetics,* 1972, 2, 262–273.

Merrill, M. D. Taxonomics, classifications, and theory. In R. N. Singer (ed.), *The psychomotor domain: movement behaviors.* Philadelphia: Lea & Febiger, 1972.

Miller, R. B. Task taxonomy: science or technology? *Ergonomics,* 1967, 10, 167–176.

Poulton, E. C. On prediction in skilled movements. *Psychological Bulletin,* 1957, 54, 467–478.

Simpson, E. J. The classification of educational objectives: psychomotor domain. *Illinois Teacher of Home Economics,* 1966–1967, 10, 110–144.

Singer, R. N. and Dick, W. *Teaching physical education: a systems approach,* second edition. Boston: Houghton Mifflin, 1980.

Singer, R. N. and Gerson, R. F. Task classification of strategy utilization in motor skills. *Research Quarterly for Exercise and Sport,* 1981, 52, 100–116.

Singer, R. N., Milne, C., Magill, R., Powell, F. M., and Vachon, L. *Laboratory and field experiment in motor learning.* Springfield, Ill.: Charles C Thomas, 1975.

5

THE ACQUISITION
OF SKILL

The primary objective in motor learning situations is to learn a movement activity. The study of motor learning is also the study of how skill is acquired, what influences its attainment, and perhaps how it is retained over time.

In this chapter we will attempt to give meaning, other than the obvious, to the term *skill*. Skill has *relative* and *absolute* properties. It can be considered on a relative basis; that is, it can refer to one's achievement in an activity relative to the achievements of others or against norms. Then again, definite hierarchical criteria for skill level may be determined for a particular task, in which case one's level of skill is defined by a standard of reference. Examples in a sport are scoring systems devised for gymnastics and diving.

Characteristics and properties of skill relative to activities and objectives will be explained. The characteristics of beginners will be analyzed, too. Stages in learning and in general what happens during learning will be discussed. Next, the ability to predict ultimate success on the basis of initial skill and characteristics will be analyzed. The chapter is concluded with an exploration of factors that contribute to differences among learners in their ability to learn specific activities and activities in general. One of those factors concerns developmental and maturational considerations. The physical readiness to learn—anything—is a very important factor in instructional settings. Now let us revisit *skill* and gain a greater understanding of its characteristics.

WHAT IS SKILL?

As we practice at an activity, evaluations are occurring continuously. We can assess present performance against previous performance. Thus we can observe a measure of improvement, which is an indication of learning, of progress, of the *process* of skill attainment.

A comparison of our performances against those of others or against normative standards indicates level of skill, but in a different context. The types of information derived from comparisons to self and to others are different. Likewise, motivation may be influenced differentially under each condition. Certain students seem to thrive under peer-competitive conditions. Other students are frustrated and become anxious. They prefer a self-evaluation approach.

Regardless of assessment technique,[1] certain parameters of performance seem to change with the learning of an activity:

(1) *Objectives* and *criteria* are closer to being realized. Higher-level objectives and criteria—that are potentially attainable—necessitate a display of greater performance (skill).

(2) *Mechanical* (habit-like) or *adaptive behaviors* are expressed appropriately depending on the activity and the situation.

(3) More *self-controlling* and directional factors operate; less external control and dependency on others.

(4) Performance becomes more *stable, consistent,* and *predictable.*

(5) Performance is more *efficient* and *effortless.*

(6) *Form,* if necessary, is more consistent with expectations.

In other words, with learning movement production appears more as it should; as it is expected to be; processes and abilities are used more effectively. Most skilled performers have learned not only how to execute acts, but also how to optimize motivational and arousal states, attention, concentration, and decision-making. Thus skill is the ability to perform an act or activity well within any situational context. When we analyze the characteristics of "typical" beginning learners, it becomes apparent what has to be overcome to progress.

---

[1] You may want to re-read Chapter 3 on techniques to measure learning. The assumption is that as learning occurs, skill is improved. The assessment of motor learning level is often the assessment of skill level, and typical parameters of behavior were described in Chapter 3.

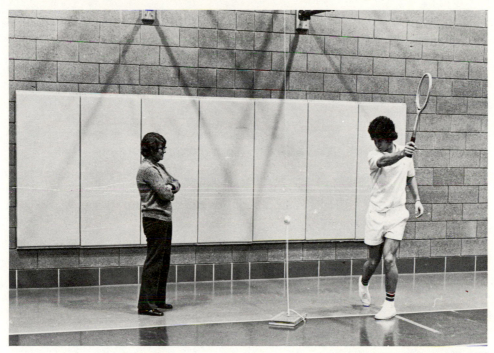

Featherkill Studios, Burnsville, MN

Tennis contains many elements of difficulty, and the instructor can simplify the information processing and movement demands placed on the learner.

CHARACTERISTICS OF BEGINNERS

When attempts to acquire skill are made, the more complex the demands, the more challenges and frustrations we presume that the learner may suffer through. Yet we all, in a relative sense, can and do succeed in certain endeavors. We don't in others. Why?

Trace your own efforts and outcomes. Pick a movement activity: sport, dance, or something else. Why did you do well in, or at least pretty well at, one activity? What factors contributed? What did you have to overcome? How long did it take before you were satisfied with your performance? Were you ever really satisfied?

Pick another activity, one you did not do well in. Analyze the circumstances. What factors operated to work against you? Could you have achieved—if you really wanted to? If yes, why didn't you? If no, why not?

We are complex, so complex. And so many activities appear complex to us that we might learn. In reality, a good portion of our problem may center around attitudes, anxiety, frustrations, coping abilities, and other personal factors that can *influence* our rate and level of achievement. A beginner, child or adult, is influenced by level of physical conditioning to practice, attitudes, emotions, expectations, past experiences, and cognitive and movement-mechanics capabilities.

Since people differ in so many ways, it is not easy to describe characteristics in common among learners. However, let's give it a try. Beginners tend:

(1) to be *attentive* to *too many cues* in a situation. They need to learn to be more selective; to attend to the minimum but most relevant cues in a situation at any given time.

(2) to *think* and *worry* too much, about too many things. A state of *relaxed concentration* for learning and performance is the desired goal.

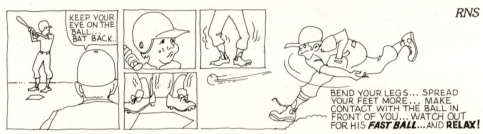

RNS

Reprinted by permission of the American Alliance for Health, Physical Education, Recreation and Dance, 1900 Association Drive, Reston VA 22091.

(3) to lack the ability to set *realistic expectations* for themselves in performance—sometimes they are too high, other times too low.

(4) to have difficulties with *too much information* (instructions and directions) given to them at one time. Teachers and coaches are often guilty of providing *information overload:* overloading the minds of learners.

(5) to view each learning experience as truly new. Yet, in reality, new learnings are derived from old learnings. Gross movement patterns, such as throwing and kicking, serve as the basis of more complex ball sports skills. *Relationships* of already acquired skills to newly introduced ones need to be perceived.

(6) to lack appropriate *strategies* to handle information and situations.

(7) to lack the knowledge of when and how to use available response-produced *feedback*.

(8) to lack *confidence* and *security;* they need positive experiences.

(9) to expend too much *unnecessary energy.*

In subsequent chapters we will deal with instructional and practice conditions that can help to overcome these problems.

A beginner obviously is a beginner owing to lack of direct experience in the activity to be learned. The mechanics of the movements need to be acquired and refined. What to do, and when, comes with experience and good guidance. Assuming appropriate physical conditioning, attitudes, and motivation on the part of the learner, and quality practice conditions and guidance from the teacher, a beginner should not remain a beginner for long.

Remember, there are differences among learners, and each responds to the learning situation in his or her own way. In many ways, children and beginning adult learners are similar in how they approach learning activities, but they differ in some important ways. We will examine student differences at the end of this chapter, and the implications for teaching.

Remember also that each motor activity makes unique demands on students. Activity classification systems were discussed in the last chapter. If we simply

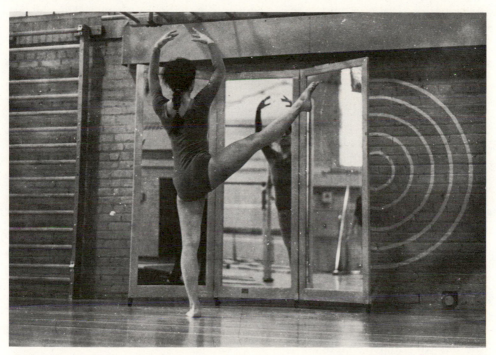

Featherkill Studios, Burnsville, MN

The acquisition of skill requires dedicated and persistent practice.

re-examine the nature of open (externally-paced) and closed (self-paced) tasks, it becomes apparent that beginners will need to develop distinct strategies for the learning/performance of each type. In closed tasks, like hitting a golf ball, tremendous concentration skills and mechanically-perfected movements are needed. By contrast, in continuous basketball play, the ability to anticipate and think ahead are valuable assets. Here both mechanically sound skills and adaptive behaviors are needed, and decision-making may have to occur in a fraction of a second.

It is felt that learners go through stages, from novice to proficient. We will discuss characteristics of the highly skilled in Chapter 9. At that time, we will make many comparisons between the relatively skilled and relatively unskilled. Not only is this information interesting but it is also suggestive of instructional considerations compatible with the skill level of performers. For now, typical stages, or phases, that learners undergo with practice will be discussed.

STAGES IN LEARNING

As a person practices and learns, changes occur. Some changes are obvious, others subtle. Sometimes they appear dramatically, but usually they are slow and gradual. Skills, strategies, and psychological-support processes are developed.

Do you remember when and how you first learned to play basketball? You probably had observed good players, in person or on television. You may have received verbal instruction. Then you tried to dribble a ball. Or to shoot it at the basket.

As you attempted one of these acts, say dribbling, so many things were on your mind. You had to look at the ball as you dribbled it. You tried to remember what you saw, what you heard, as to the techniques involved in the task. The ball seemed so difficult, if not impossible, to control, especially as you attempted to walk, then run, while dribbling. You concentrated on the ball and the act of bouncing it. Finally, you got the idea of what needed to be done and how to do it.

Then either you were instructed or you figured out for yourself how to practice dribbling. What conditions seemed to be most favorable to improvement? For example, did you attempt to continually practice the activity for one period of time in a day (massed practice), or did you space practice throughout the day (distributed practice)?

After sufficient practice, you were able to dribble as if it were a subconscious act. You did not have to look at the ball. You could run, dribble, shoot, or even think of playing strategy *while* dribbling. You had achieved the highest level of skill: automaticity. In other words, dribbling could occur without deliberate consciousness of the act.

Paul Fitts and Michael Posner (1967) have identified three stages that would describe the dribbling example or the learning of any motor skill. In reality, learning is a continuous process. The stages are identified and characterized as a matter of convenience, to highlight occurrences at the beginning, middle, and final phases in the development of skill:

(1) *The cognitive phase* occurs *early* in learning. The student makes attempts at understanding the nature of the activity to be learned. Thought processes are heavily involved at this stage. The student has to understand the intention and purposes of certain motor acts, analyze the situation, and devise techniques to fulfill goals. The student also has to convert verbal directions in to meaningful movement behaviors. This may be more of a problem than most people realize. Children don't always understand "adult" words and descriptions. Ethnic and cultural differences between teacher and student may also lead to communication

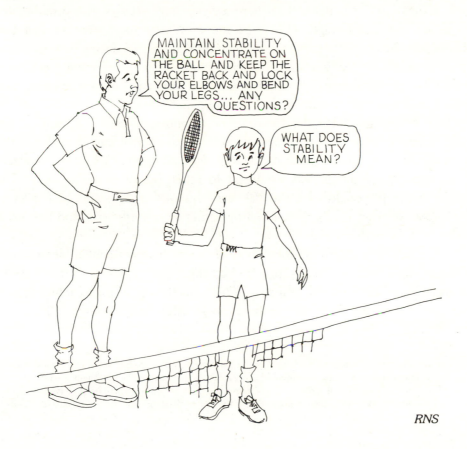

RNS

breakdowns between them, when the teacher's explanations of what is to be learned are not comprehended by the students.

(2) *The associative phase* is *intermediate* between beginning and highest levels of skill. At this stage, the learner understands what needs to be done; the concern is now for correct practice techniques that will promote the learning of the activity. There are many questions about ideal practice techniques and conditions. We will address many of them in subsequent chapters, such as: Is it better to emphasize speed in the learning of a movement? Or is accuracy (form) more important? Should a skill be practiced in its entirety? Should it be practiced in parts? Is it more desirable to distribute practice over time? Or is a large amount of practice at one time more effective?

(3) The *autonomous* phase is considered the *final* one in the process of acquiring skill. At this level, the performer is able to process information easily, with minimal interference from other ongoing activities. The behavior is automatic; there is minimal conscious control over the movement.

As was mentioned before, there is convenience in noting distinct stages in the learning of a skill. Whereas Fitts and Posner describe three such stages, Jack Adams (1971)[2] believes that there are two major stages: the verbal-motor stage and the motor stage. The *verbal-motor stage* is similar to the first two phases described by Fitts and Posner. Much thinking occurs during early learning. Many decisions are being made concerning strategies and movement mechanics. Variability in movement is very noticeable. Consistency in performance and refined skill are associated with the second or motor stage.

As is the case with the Fitts-Posner autonomous phase, Adams' *motor stage* is associated with automaticity. There is self-control and direction, little need of help from others. Automaticity in performing one task frees the attentional capacity of the person to attend to other things simultaneously. The skilled soccer player dribbles the ball with his or her feet and at the same time is considering field strategies, anticipating where offensive and defensive players will be within moments.

A completely different orientation of research offers similar descriptions of the learning process and of progress in reaching proficiency, with implications for instruction. Research on human *abilities*, and their relation to achievements in a task at different stages of practice, reveals interesting findings.

---

[2] Actually Adams' article is very important reading for the serious student of motor learning. Besides describing stages in learning, he addressed issues concerning the control of movement. Many arguments have been offered as to the notion of central (program) control versus peripheral (feedback) control of movement. We will talk more about this in the chapter dealing with the highly skilled.

ABILITIES AND THEIR RELATIONSHIP TO SKILL

Before we summarize the findings on abilities and success, it would be wise first to clarify terminology that has been used somewhat interchangeably by the average person.

A *skill, task*, or *activity* usually refers to a specific set of responses that is to be made in a particular situation in which there are criteria, standards, and expectations in performance.

Theoretically, an *ability* is a trait. Its presence, at an ideal level, underlies or contributes to success in a number of related skills. An ability is not a specific act, as a skill is. Rather, it is usually thought to be an enduring quality, a personal characteristic affected by both genetics and experience. By contrast, a skill is learned.

Edwin Fleishman (1975) and his colleagues have studied the nature of abilities for many years. A number of abilities have been identified, as has their relationship to the acquisition of skill. Most importantly, it has been noted that:

(1) a *greater number* of abilities (more general to the task) contribute to learning a task in the early stages than do so later on.

(2) *different* and *fewer* abilities (more task-specific) contribute more and more to success with practice.

Let us consider these findings for a moment, from a practical perspective. Once again, we are reminded of the importance of activity analysis (see Chapter 4 again). When we realize the kinds of demand that activities make on students, we can determine what kinds of ability are needed to succeed in them. And, as students become more skilled at what they are doing, different kinds of ability will contribute to achievement. The sensitive teacher emphasizes the use of the appropriate abilities through proper cuing and training techniques.

For example, verbal comprehension as an ability is very important at the earliest stage of learning when directions are given from a teacher to a student. An inability to understand directions or to translate words into movements precludes the possibility of effective movement. At this stage too, more general abilities, like spatial orientation and balance, are important. As the learner acquires skill, fewer and more task-specific abilities play a dominant role.

See if you can analyze a sport such as volleyball. Determine the kinds of abilities that might be important to a volleyball player. Which abilities appear to be more important at the earliest stage, for a beginner? Which seems more important at the intermediate level? Which are of primary importance to the skilled volleyball player?

FROM EXTERNAL TO SELF-CONTROL

Basically, an analysis of stages, abilities, or other factors suggests that when it means to be skilled is to be able to perform more under *one's own control* than under the control of situations and other people (teachers, coaches). Self-control holds many implications.

On one hand, it means being able to analyze situations and tasks for oneself, knowing quickly what to do and how to do it. It means needing very little feedback from others about performance execution; knowing what to pay attention to during performance and when, what and how to analyze after the performance is over. On the other hand, it means the ability to control one's emotions, attitudes, concentration, and other psychological processes supportive of and associated with achievement in motor skills.

The challenge to the learner and the instructor is to develop means by which the learner can become a more self-sufficient, independent learner and performer. It is little wonder that Tim Gallwey's books, e.g., *The Inner Game of Tennis* (1974) have become so popular. He has attempted to analyze the psychological processes that the highly skilled use, and to have beginners do the same. He is a strong advocate of "letting the body do its thing," thinking as little as possible during performance ("quieting the mind"), putting oneself in a state of "relaxed concentration," and in general, thinking positively of one's capabilities.

PREDICTING ACHIEVEMENT

We all like to guess at the achievement potential of beginners in an activity. Consider a class of children taking gymnastics for the first time. On the basis of initial performance, we might attempt to predict which children will be the most successful at the end of the unit of instruction. What is the basis for these predictions? In fact, how accurate will they be?

Some expert baseball coaches say that they can tell right away if a ballplayer is a ballplayer. Maury Willis, upon taking over the management of a professional baseball team in midsummer of 1980, stated "It will take me only a day to tell who's a player. Watch a player run once or twice, and you can tell if he is or has the potential to steal bases."

Many teachers make the same claims. Very often students are placed in groups on the basis of similar abilities or skills. Homogenous groupings of students may be easier to teach than an extremely heterogeneous group with diverse capabilities. Of course, when under-expectations for achievements are made— by the teacher or by the student—there is always the danger of the *self-fulfilling prophecy*. That is, people tend to behave or perform as they think they are expected to. That's okay with high expectations. But low expectations? Well . . .

Predicting achievement is not as easy as it sounds. Motor learning research will attest to this. One technique is to determine skill level for a group of subjects in a task on an initial trial or block of trials. Then a number of practice trials is administered. The subjects are then officially tested again. Will those subjects who performed the best initially also be those who are the highest achievers at the end of practice and vice versa?

On the basis of (1) *limited observations,* (2) a *complex task,* and (3) *long duration of practice,* accurate predictions are difficult to make. This is especially true the more alike in skill a group is at the start of a learning experience. Some research (e.g., Welch and Henry, 1971) indicates that about 50 per cent of the scores, or one-half of practice is necessary before meaningful predictions of relative achievement can be established.

If a task is relatively *simple,* and practice duration is not long, predictions are easier. This is probably because fewer capabilities are necessary to achieve the task. Learners become more alike quickly, although relative initial differences remain somewhat the same at the end of practice. On the basis of motor learning research, then, the predictiveness of early performance for later performance in a task depends on a number of factors.

Speaking of predictions, the ability to predict athletic potential from childhood to adolescence is of great interest in many countries. When attempting to train would-be world-class athletes, it would be ideal to know which youngsters have the potential to realize success if given extensive training. In the Soviet Union and sister countries, children are selected on the basis of many types of tests for special training in sport and dance. Research is lacking on gifted performers and accuracy of predicting skill attainment, however.

Yet school athletes have been studied longitudinally in this country. G. Lawrence Rarick (1980) has summarized much of the research on motor development. In reporting prediction data, he states that it is extremely hazardous to predict athletic achievement from elementary school to junior high school. Only one-quarter of a sample of subjects were considered outstanding in both types of schools. Rarick suggests that "the reason for such ability shift may well be as much a function of changing interests as a reflection of changes in basic performance capabilities" (p. 59).

GENERAL ABILITY CONCEPTS: FACT OR FICTION?

"What a genius!" "What a gifted person!" "What a natural athlete!" Expressions like these heard all the time, reflecting a common opinion of the generality of personal qualities. But let's explore this area further. It's filled with misconceptions.

General Motor Ability Tests

When the IQ test was developed early in this century to predict intelligence and potential to achieve academically, it is little wonder that physical educators attempted the same in their field: to develop tests to predict the ability to achieve in sports. They fell far short of the mark.

A typical motor ability test contained three to seven skills tests. The test predicted best to those sports which contained these kinds of skill. But mostly, it seemed as if there were no such thing as a general motor ability. There are *many motor abilities*, the exact number of which is unknown. Different activities require different abilities, and in various combinations. Likewise, many types of intelligence exist. Creativity, problem-solving, rote memory, speed reading, and other forms of intelligence do not correlate highly with each other. There is no one mental ability.

Memory Drum Theory and Task Specificity

More than anyone concerned with motor skills and physical education, Franklin Henry, Professor Emeritus at the University of California, researched and wrote in support of the notion of task specificity. In other words, he believed that the ability to be proficient in an activity was a unique experience; there was no assurance of achieving at the same level in other activities.

Henry's ideas are best expressed in the October issue of *The Research Quarterly* (1960), in which he proposed his "Memory Drum Theory." Basically, he suggested that acts we learn are stored in our memory system, like a computer's, in specific grooves. When acts are very closely related, transfer possibilities are greater. Much of the research completed by him and his colleagues was undertaken on acts requiring fast reactions or speed of limb movement. Speed was not found to be a unitary factor. In other words, a person who was fast at one movement was not necessarily fast with another movement. These reaction time/movement time studies provided heavy support for the notion of task specificity.

All-Round Athlete

As we can refute the notion of the existence of a general motor ability, or a generality factor that allows one person to succeed in all sorts of endeavors, one can also question whether there are many all-round athletes. True, some individuals can and do succeed in a number of activities. But this is the exception, not the rule.

To the extent that similar equipment, skills, and strategies are involved in different activities, there is a better chance for an athlete in one sport to succeed in another one. Of course, motivation and need to achieve are important variables, too. All too often much is expected from an athlete who has achieved well in one sport as to how he or she will perform in a "new" sport.

Skill, or extremely high competence, in highly complex activities, takes a long time to develop. Both heredity and intensive training produce performances at the highest level. Athletes who are successful in a number of sports, have probably practiced in a committed manner in each of these sports, especially if these sports are unrelated in the demands they impose on the performer.

The Relationship of Cognitive and Motor Abilities

The concept of mind and body united, as one, is old and true. Our behaviors reflect the interaction of the two. To what degree the ability to achieve in motor skills is related to success in so-called intellectual endeavors is a question not necessarily answered as easily as the belief in the relationship of mind and body.

In the "normal" population of people, one cannot predict success in motor skills on the basis of intellectual test scores, or vice versa. This is true with outstanding athletes. It is also true with those who are classified as geniuses.

The only group of people in which there is a reasonable relationship between cognitive and motor capabilities is the *mentally retarded*. Retarded youngsters appear to be two to four years behind in motor development as compared to similar-aged normal students. Special instructional materials and approaches have been prepared for the retarded to teach them both academic matter and motor skills.

INDIVIDUAL DIFFERENCES

The study of abilities and characteristics reveals that students differ in many ways. Furthermore, they will not all respond to the same instruction in the same way. They possess dissimilar abilities and capabilities, will learn at varying rates, and will demonstrate relative achievement as a function of a multitude of factors.

In the preceding sections on "predicting the attainment of skill" and "general ability concepts," many popular notions were disputed. Proficiency in complex motor skills depends on the interplay of many variables. We casually make statements about people, and assume the "generality" of factors and accomplishments. But proficiency in a complex activity does not come easy. It reflects personal capabilities brought to the learning situation and associated with both potential to accomplish the task and persistent practice at it.

Even the ability to learn quickly or slowly is not necessarily a general characteristic of an individual but probably is related more to the nature of the task. Thus a person may be a relatively fast learner in swimming and a relatively slow learner in racketball. Learners differ not only in rate of learning in a particular task, but also in their motivation and strategies and techniques for learning.

The recognition of such differences in learners with regard to achievement in educational programs has encouraged a philosophy dedicated to more individualized learning programs. A book by L. J. Cronbach and R. E. Snow (1977) is recommended for those of you who wish to read an overview of research on the relationship of aptitudes, abilities, and learning styles to various instructional approaches and potential techniques to improve learner performance. The general premise is that a particular type of instructional method is more appropriate than others for certain learners.

FORM

Of the many ways students may differ in the learning and performance of a motor activity, one is in *form*, the personal expression of movement. It is usually a poor idea for a beginner or even an advanced learner to copy every phase of an act from someone else. Differences in body size, personalities, and other factors indicate the undesirability of attempting to duplicate the form of another in every aspect of an activity.

Although forms may vary, even among great athletes in the same sport, it is rare when they violate established performance principles. In any skill, there is probably generally accepted biomechanical evidence for its execution,

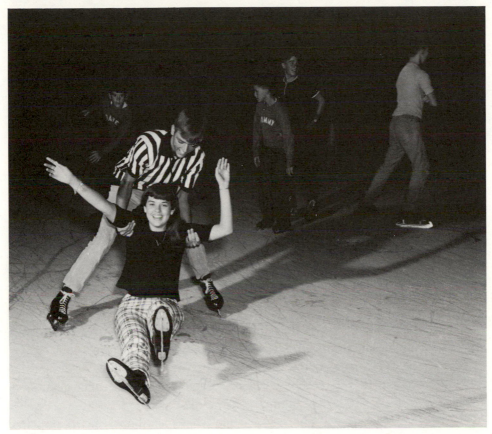

Photo by Cindy Brown

Learning can be fun.

with acceptable variations of the ideal form. In sports like gymnastics, figure skating, and diving, judgments are made on skill and form. In most sports, the outcome is more important than the means. When people attempt to acquire skills, they are usually taught "optimal form." However, due to great differences in body structure and condition, alternative movement possibilities exist in the realization of skilled performance.

READINESS TO LEARN

In this chapter we have dealt with many considerations about people, people who are in the beginning stages of attempting to learn a skill. Of all the factors involved, one of the most important is readiness and willingness. Readiness can be interpreted in several ways.

Motivation and Attitude

Readiness to learn can refer to a student's *receptivity* to instructions, programs, and goals. The learning environment must be conducive to learning. The teacher's impression on and communication with students are extremely important. In other words, the student's frame of mind toward the learning activity will make a big difference in achievement and enjoyment. Motivational techniques will be dealt with in a later chapter.

Arousal State

The learner's state of arousal *(emotions)* is related to his or her learning and performance potential. Emotions need to be *optimal*—for the person and the activity—for best results.

The best athletes have learned to control and direct their thoughts and feelings, prior to and during performance. Unfortunately, the processes involved are rarely taught by coaches. Some athletes just seem to figure them out, to problem-solve. Yet, many don't. Many students in classes, too, have learning problems because they have not developed *coping skills*, the management of anxiety, of pressure, of fear of failure, and the like.

Effective teachers will observe students whose learning is being impaired due to emotional and attitudinal problems. These problems need to be overcome. A student may want badly to learn to swim, but be afraid of the water. Swimming skills are not difficult to learn, except when emotional blocks are present. Such is the case with all motor activities. Too little or too much motivation or emotions may impair learning/performance.

DEVELOPMENTAL CONSIDERATIONS

Most of you will probably deal with children in in-school and out-of-school physical education, athletic, and recreational programs. There is much that you need to know about developmental and maturational readiness to learn and perform skills. Children often have a greater capacity than expected to do well in a variety of athletic events. They have limitations as well. Let us explore their capabilities further.

Children as Beginners

In many ways, children learning motor skills should be considered in the same way as adult beginners. But among differences to consider between adults and children are:

(1) *The development of the nervous and musculature systems.* The learning of specific sports skills will be hindered the more the child is developmentally immature.

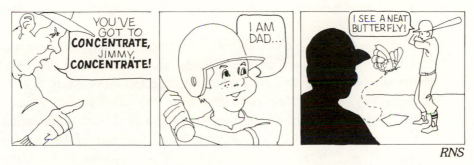

RNS

Reprinted by permission of the American Alliance for Health, Physical Education, Recreation and Dance, 1900 Association Drive, Reston, VA 22091.

(2) *Background experiences.* The adult has a richer and varied background of experiences; the child is much more limited. This can work to the advantage of disadvantage of either. Consider that what we have experienced and learned before helps *(positive transfer)* or hampers *(negative transfer)* present learnings.

There are many activities that children seem to learn much faster than adults. They have not developed inhibitions, fears, and the wrong response tendencies. (Note how easily children learn foreign languages. They have not as yet developed a strong repertoire of English words and are often more adept than adults at acquiring words and meanings in other languages.)

Then again, adults can apply many previous learning experiences to newly-introduced ones. When closely allied, the past experiences can facilitate the acquisition of new learnings.

(3) *Communication fluency.* Since adults are usually the teachers and coaches of others, child learners may be at a disadvantage as compared to adult learners. Children's verbal and comprehension skills are lower; their attention span is more limited.

(4) *Ability to endure practice sessions.* Practice can be monotonous and boring—for anyone. Since a child's span of attention is typically more limited than that of an adult, repetitive practice routines and drills may deter motivation and enthusiasm.

In general, children are restless and active. Your challenge is to maintain their enthusiasm for sport, play, and exercise, offer adequate guidance, and get as many students as possible immersed in activity. With regard to instruction, consider:

(1) *Fun.* Why not make learning situations enjoyable as well as productive? Learning drills can be made into games. Adults have learned to discipline themselves in order to work hard to attain goals; children have not.

(2) *Communication.* Be clear, specific, and brief in what you want your students to do. Don't assume that the child has already developed the ability to associate verbal labels for expected movements.

(3) *Being positive.* Negative comments from the teacher lead to lower self-concepts, frustration, and a wish to be removed from the situation. Encouragement and a positive attitude on the part of the teacher will influence the child's attitudes toward participation and achievement in physical activity.

(4) *Reinforcement.* Reinforcement can be derived from one's own interpretation of a performance or by feedback from someone else. In either case, an evaluation of performance in terms of being successful or failing, good or bad, is important in an activity. Consequently, greater efforts should be made to encourage kids to compare their performance with their own previous ones rather than with the performance of others. Many times kids perform well but lose in a contest. Their performance may have improved over the last time, yet they are criticized and dejected for losing when they played well. Self-competition can lead to a greater probability of reinforcement for more participants.

(5) *Information processing deficits.* Children need to learn the appropriate strategies to manage information and make accurate as well as quick decisions. They lack experience. They must learn to develop their capacities—and they will—with sensitive and meaningful guidance.

There are so many other developmental factors to consider, and we will consider them shortly for all learners. For now, just remember that one of your major roles as a teacher is to help *all* children learn skills, knowledges, and favorable attitudes related to physical activity. Start with the philosophy that

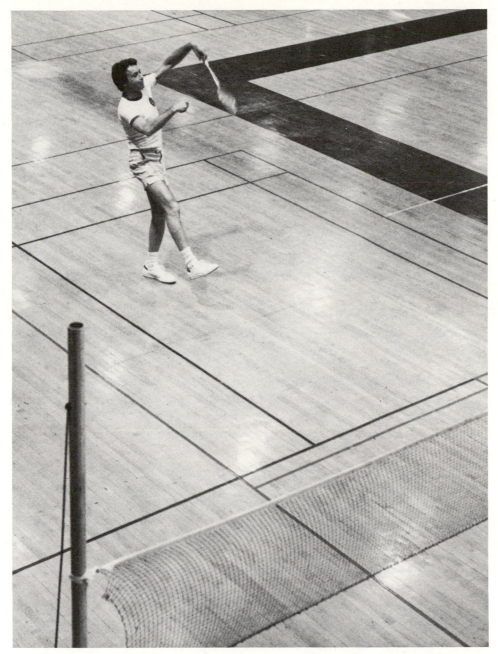

City News Bureau, St. Petersburg, Flordia

The left-handed form displayed by the author, which has led him to many local, regional, and national defeats in badminton! In this case, form might improve execution.

every child deserves to learn and to improve. You can promote this process if you are knowledgeable about the activity and about children, and how to communicate with them.

SUMMARY

The ease and effectiveness of acquiring skill depends on a host of biomechanical, physiological, psychological, and sociological factors, as well as on the teacher's understanding and communication capabilities. Beginners go through stages in the learning process, with different abilities playing different roles as skill is acquired. Once skill is attained, the person seems to possess control and direction over his or her actions and personal states, and performance level is high, consistent, and somewhat predictable.

Predicting later achievement in motor skills is not easy. One way is to use initial scores on the particular skill. It was shown that this approach is only effective if the skill is easy to learn, practice time brief, and the subjects heterogeneous in performance in that skill at the beginning of practice. Otherwise, a considerable number of practice scores and sessions will be required for adequate prediction.

The notion of the existence of general ability has been misleading in many ways. First of all, tests that presumably measure general motor ability do not predict achievement very well in most sports. Anyway, there is probably no such thing as general motor ability or general athletic ability. Rather, many abilities exist, and the presence of some to an ideal degree help to contribute to success in a particular skill. The extent to which our capabilities can generalize across situations and learning tasks or are uniquely specific has been argued about throughout this century. Some generalization is possible, but more complex skills require more task-specific practice and capabilities.

Students differ in a variety of characteristics meaningful for learning and performance. When it is possible, alternative instructional approaches can help more learners than can one approach for all. The readiness to learn was discussed as an important prerequisite for learning. Developmental readiness and special considerations for youthful beginning learners were areas elaborated upon. Children *must* receive quality, meaningful, and enjoyable learning experiences if they are to remain interested in participating and achieving at motor skills.

REFERENCES AND SUGGESTED READINGS

Adams, J. A. A closed-loop theory of motor learning. *Journal of Motor Behavior,* 1971, 3, 111–150.

Connolly, K. The nature of motor skill development. *Journal of Human Movement Studies,* 1977, 3, 128–143.

Cronbach, L. J. and Snow, R. E. *Aptitudes and instructional methods: a handbook for research on interactions.* New York: Irvington, 1977.

Fitts, P. M. and Posner, M. I. *Human performance.* Belmont, Cal.: Brooks/Cole, 1967, Chapter 2.

Fleishman, E. A. Toward a taxonomy of human performance. *American Psychologist,* 1975, 30, 1127–1149.

Gallwey, W. T. *The inner game of tennis.* New York: Random House, 1974.

Henry, F. M. Increased response latency for complicated movements and a "memory drum" theory of neuromotor reaction. *Research Quarterly,* 1960, 31, 448–458.

Rarick, G. L. Motor development: its growing knowledge base. *Journal of Physical Education and Recreation,* 1980, 51, 26–27, 56–59, 61.

Welch, M. and Henry, F. M. Individual differences in various parameters. *Journal of Motor Behavior,* 1971, 3, 78–96.

6

ESTABLISHING PRACTICE CONDITIONS

After reading the previous chapter, we now have a feeling for the common characteristics of beginners as well as the characteristics wherein they may differ. The theorist is *descriptive* whereas the teacher or coach is expected to be *prescriptive*. Practice conditions, when well planned, should lead beginners to reasonably skilled levels as painlessly and efficiently as possible.

Instructional design is the formal, systematic planning of teaching in a particular situation. As a doctor might prescribe drugs for an ailing patient, the teacher is expected to be able to prescribe appropriate learning procedures and conditions for students. In this chapter, we will discuss systems models for instruction and their role in instructional design.

Practice is at the heart of improvement. Many factors must be considered when practice conditions are being planned. Sometimes there are tradeoffs: something gained for something lost. Sometimes certain conditions are thought to be beneficial for all participants in a program. Then again, alternative modes may be equally effective in helping different types of learners achieve the same goals. Group-oriented and individualized (with the use of media) instruction will be analyzed and compared. By the end of this chapter, I hope you will appreciate the great importance of practice considerations and the role a teacher can play in facilitating the learning process.

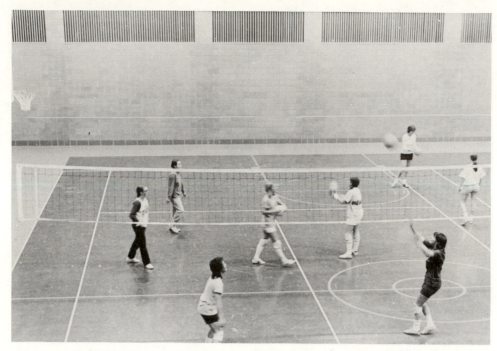

Featherkill Studios, Burnsville, MN

Practice does not always have to involve the same repetitive drills for beginners.

THE DESIGN OF INSTRUCTION

Instruction can be a science. One develops blueprints for making things, lesson plans, or training program plans to promote learning. Carefully thought out plans, consistent with scientific evidence as to the nature of learners and learning environments, should lead to a higher probability of successful outcomes. Increased concern for and consideration of the science of instruction has been shown by many leading educational psychologists, such as Robert Glaser (1976). His article is excellent background reading on this topic.

Thus, as stated before, instructional design (the blueprint for instruction) should not be taken lightly. The process of acquiring skill—in anything—presents a challenge. Major and minor problems have to be solved by both the learner and the teacher. Some of the problems that beginners face were described briefly in the previous chapter. Many more characteristics of learners and obstacles that learners have to overcome to achieve skill and satisfaction could have been identified. The fact that complex acts, as performed in sports, are not mastered easily indicates the significant role that the well-prepared and qualified instructor can and should play in the guidance offered to students.

This is why you must:

(1) analyze carefully the skills and activities that are to be taught, considering the ideal sequence of events to achieve your objectives.

(2) analyze sensitively the children under your direction, in order to become aware of the general behavioral and skill characteristics of the group as well as noting meaningful individual differences.

(3) attempt to apply information learned in this book and other books, in this class and other classes, to the way you design instruction and communicate with students.

A systematic analysis of tasks, situations, and goals suggests a scientific and important approach in instruction. Every student deserves to learn and to improve. You can facilitate this process if you are knowledgeable about the activity and the children you are teaching, about how to communicate with them, and about how to plan class or practice sessions effectively.

SYSTEMS APPROACHES

The word *system* is used quite frequently. Physiologically oriented discussions will include reference to the digestive, nervous, and circulatory systems. Computer and machine systems include a network of mechanisms constructed for an expressed purpose. The teacher and the coach have formulated systems under which they and their students will work. Systems, whether they refer to machinery, person-machine interactions, or human functioning and behavior, include purposes, systems parts, and relationships.

The system usually connotes a "wholeness." That is, the system is the entire functioning unit, complete with subsystems, that works together to fulfill some objective. However, there are many examples of systems within systems; that is, a system may be complete when viewed one way and yet be part of a larger system. A person's behavior, as represented by a response made to a situation, could be examined systematically and referred to as a behavioral system, or it could be examined within the context of an organized sport activity. The system is thereby enlarged, more variables are viewed, and the arrangement becomes more complex and intricately woven. Look at the educational system, which contains as subsystems an administrative system, a purchasing system, an instructional system, and many others. If the school system is to work, all of its component systems (subsystems) must operate interrelatedly at high levels of capability. The same is true of organized sports, for similar reasons.

Systems Models for Instruction

Systems analysis helps to define the series of operations and the involvement of the varous parts contributing to the objective. On this level, such an analysis merely states the obvious. But it often happens that obvious procedures are not followed or are followed poorly. The systematic approach to studying human behavior requires the identification of contributing units and how they interact to influence learning and performance. The meaning of the analysis is enhanced as scientific rigor is applied. Systems analysis provides a means for examining human behavior in an organized, dynamic manner, whereby links are identified and interdependently expressed, as research and theory permit. Decision making in practical situations, knowledge of what behavior needs to be applied, and information description based on scientific knowledge are all enhanced by systems

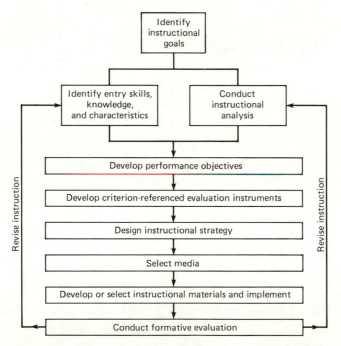

Figure 6–1. Systems approach model for instruction. (From R. N. Singer and W. Dick, *Teaching Physical Education: A Systems Approach.* 2d ed. Boston: Houghton Mifflin, 1980.)

analysis. The systems approach is a way (not the only one, but certainly one of the more popular today) of thinking of entire operations and their component parts. Beyond description, it is an effective approach in instruction to examining alternatives and making decisions, as emphasized by Singer (1977).

Systems design experts have been active in industry, the military, and, more recently, in education. Robert N. Singer and Walter Dick (1980) have proposed a systems model that can be used in instruction, and they have developed systems materials expressly for the teaching of physical education. Figure 6–1 contains the complete instructional system model. It suggests a flow of activities that a teacher would conduct in order to produce effective instruction. There are many instructional models in use today; all have many similarities and differ primarily in certain components or in the sequence in which the components are diagrammed.

Instructional analysis should proceed in a systematic way. A specific but partial analysis is made in Figure 6–2, where a hierarchy of skills is indicated for the learner to achieve the objective of effectively participating in a nine-inning baseball game. A task analysis must be made in order to determine the

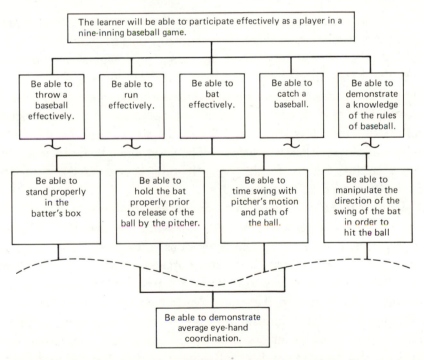

Figure 6–2. Example of a partial learning hierarchy resulting from an instructional analysis. (From R. N. Singer and W. Dick, *Teaching Physical Education: A Systems Approach,* 2d ed. Boston: Houghton Mifflin, 1980.)

subordinate tasks prerequisite for the mastery of higher-level tasks. The process of specifying the tasks and indicating their relationships in order to achieve the goal suggests that instructional analysis, a component of the instructional systems model (see Figure 6–1), follows the principles of systems analysis also. These are examples of instructional systems. It is also possible to develop a system that describes human behavior.

Systems Models of Human Motor Behavior

A behaving system, be it person or machine, contains certain prerequisite characteristics. In fact, a usual reference in the psychological literature is to person-machine systems, where several human and machine components are designed to work together to fulfill some goal. Transportation systems, such as flying a plane, require the harmonious interplay of a person and a machine. In such person-machine dynamics, there is present some form of sensing device that selectively allows some messages to continue on in the system. Noise or bias (confounding, distracting) cues can be coped with and should minimally affect output.

In these systems, operations can appear as if programmed (a set of internal instructions that assume the form of a master plan), thus the reliance on memory stores where programs can be built up and stored for usage at the appropriate signal. At the same time there is flexibility in the system—an ability to adapt to changing circumstances. There are times when a master plan must be altered, and the system should possess the desired arrangement of its components to allow for control and alteration. A well-designed system should be able to fulfill its specified objectives. Effective output will be determined by internal and external control factors, that is, by its ability to process and handle a variety of stimuli by making correct responses.

A person can be considered as a system, one that selects from available cues and responds in a purposeful manner following the activation of decision-making processes. If we were to consider various categories of tasks the human being learns to perform, perhaps a variety of models would be needed. Setting aside the contrasting characteristics of tasks, a search for commonalities among them would probably lead to the model illustrated in the next chapter. That model highlights the basic human processes involved in motor learning and performance, and provides an overview of the person as a behaving system. Influences on this behaving system will be analyzed in the remainder of this book.

TEACHING AND LEARNING STRATEGIES

"Scientifically designed instruction" implies that teachers apply plans and strategies to create favorable learning environments. Learners, too, have and use strategies to learn. Sometimes they are imposed on them by teachers; at other times they are self-initiated.

Attention must be given to various considerations with regard to learners and practice (see Figure 6–3):

(1) prior to practice (readying the learners, preparing them for what is to be learned).

(2) during practice (practice conditions, teacher guidance).

(3) after practice (feedback availability, reinforcement).

General Considerations

Before any activities are actually taught, the background, physical condition, skills, and attitudes of the learners have to be ascertained. From this information, decisions about what to teach and how to teach can be made more intelligently. An analysis of the activity should be undertaken also. To summarize, general considerations are associated with

(1) student skill, condition, knowledge, interest, and attitude level.

(2) the range of student capabilities.

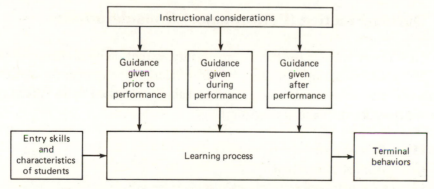

Figure 6–3. Instructional considerations in relation to performance, practice, and the learning process. (From R. N. Singer, The learning systems approach and instruction in psychomotor activities. *Motor Skills: Theory Into Practice*, 1977, 1, 113–122.)

(3) activity analysis of demands placed on the students.

(4) available resources and facilities.

Prepractice (Performance) Considerations

The major considerations here are associated with readying the learner to learn/perform and readying the learning environment so that the situation is most conducive to learning. Readying the learner has to do with

(1) establishing appropriate attitudes, motivations, and interest toward the activity.

(2) establishing rapport and good communication.

(3) explaining objectives and expected learning outcomes.

(4) communicating what the present task is (explanations, directions, student observations of the task being performed).

Mental and attitudinal readiness to learn, being receptive to what is being instructed, and understanding performance expectations are important preperformance considerations with regard to learners. The teacher's attitudes and expectations affect those of the learners. Teachers also have to make decisions about instructional settings. These include

(1) equipment and facilities

(2) special resources, such as media

(3) cues and aids that might promote learning

During-Practice (Performance) Considerations

Here our concern is for the nature, quality, extent, and conditions of practice. Many tradeoffs exist. In other words, a decision to emphasize one thing in practice may have some value as well as liability attached to it. Alternatives must be considered. Some concerns are

(1) sufficient goal-directed practice,

(2) continual motivation,

(3) appropriate sequence of activities,

(4) the distribution and scheduling of practice,

(5) fatigue and boredom, and

(6) practice methods.

How much practice is desirable depends on initial skill level and final expectations (terminal behaviors). More quality practice should lead to higher skill level. However, more practice at one activity takes away time available in class to practice something else—a tradeoff. This is an example of one of the many problems with which a teacher must wrestle.

Another problem is how to sustain the motivation of students over time. When practice becomes too routine, it becomes boring; changing practice routines helps. Being positive and showing enthusiasm helps, too; showing an interest in the progress of the students and reinforcing "the good things" that are happening both enliven the environment. Many aspects of motivation and ways to influence it will be discussed in Chapter 8.

Practice activities need to be sequenced logically; their difficulty and the relationships among these activities should be considered. The progression should be logical. The accomplishing of one task will lead to the acquisition of the next, and so on. This is a form of vertical transfer. A hierarchical arrangement of tasks from beginning to end should also be followed.

Practice schedules for a task can be relatively massed or distributed over time. An activity can be practiced in its entirety or in parts. Emphasis could be placed on speed, accuracy and form, or both in the practicing of an activity. Activities can be practiced directly (as they really exist) or under simulated (simplified) conditions. Practice can be guided very heavily with prompts and cues, or left more to the learner's problem-solving capabilities. For example, tennis strokes can be practiced one stroke at a time, with the instructor hitting the appropriate shot to the student over and over. Or students can practice against a backboard, inevitably using a variety of strokes as required.

As can be seen, many decisions need to be made as to the nature of practice and the methods used to acquire skill. A number of these considerations will be addressed shortly.

Postpractice (Performance) Considerations

Once a practice attempt, a series of attempts, or an entire practice session has been completed, consideration should be given to the type and extent of the *reinforcement* and *knowledge of results (feedback)* that it might be appropriate to provide to the student. So our immediate concerns deal with helping the learner know how well he or she is doing, from an informational and motivational perspective; and the possible need to provide both reinforcement and knowledge of results (supplementary feedback).

You probably will be concerned with more than the immediate learning/

performance of an activity. Most of the time we would like such experiences to be *remembered*. The ability to perform at a high level of skill at a later date is a function of the quality and extent of practice encountered originally. Another long-term objective has to do with *transfer*, the influence of present learnings on later learnings. Since it is impossible by teaching to prepare someone for every eventuality that might be experienced in an athletic contest or on the job, educational and training programs need to stress the learning of both fundamental skills and problem-solving (adaptive) abilities. We have been discussing *retention* in connection with basic skill learning and *transfer* in connection with adaptive abilities.

PRACTICE CONDITIONS

As we have seen from the preceding overview, many practice considerations confront the teacher of motor skills. These considerations have been highlighted to give you a feeling of what they are, and to show you that each has been an area of study in the psychology of learning. As a result of such study, we have evidence that suggests procedures that might work for most learners. Evidence exists also with regard to special considerations for different types of learners.

At this point, we are ready to explore in greater depth selected topics concerning the establishment of practice conditions.

INTRODUCING A SKILL

We have already emphasized the importance of evaluating the characteristics and skills of the learners in regard to the learning task. Instruction must begin at a level compatible with learner status. Typical approaches in introducing a skill to learners include (1) observation (viewing a live or filmed skilled performer) or (2) directions (verbal or written).

Observation

Animals observe other animals. Children observe adults and other children. Many behaviors are acquired simply through observation, without anything said. Not only are activities learned through observing and analyzing others, but so are values and all sorts of behaviors. Albert Bandura, past president of the American Psychological Association, is a foremost authority on observational learning. He has demonstrated its potential role in acquiring and modifying a large range of behaviors.

The value we intuitively give to observation has been supported by research findings; these have shown that observational learning, or the *modeling effect* (the influence of another's behavior on the behavior/performance of the observer) is very effective in learning motor skills. Better skilled models (live performers) have a more beneficial effect on learners. The frequency of the need for observational learning will depend on the complexity of the activity, the amount of practice allowed for its learning, and the perceptive abilities of the students.

Using a stabilometer, Thomas, Pierce, and Ridsdale (1977) demonstrated that second- and fourth-graders balanced better when provided with a model compared to a control group with no model. However, when the model demonstrated the skill again midway in practice, after six of the twelve allocated trials,

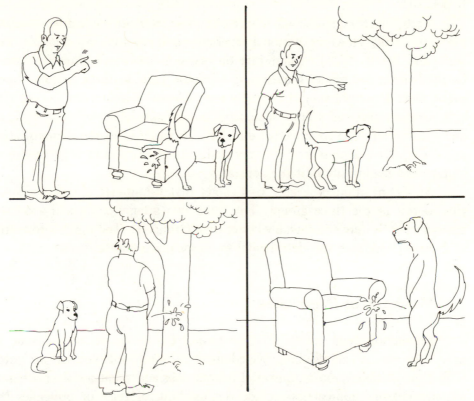

From Lefroncois, G. R.: Psychological Theories and Human Learning: Kongor's Report. *Monterey, Calif.: Brooks/Cole Publishing Co., 1972.*

only the older group was benefited. Apparently, as children get older they can process more information and use this additional information to their advantage.

Learners can get this idea of what they need to learn and to do by observing a well-performed live act. Films, slides, photographs, and other forms of media may be helpful, too. The quality of these is important. So are student receptivity, understanding, and motivation.

Verbal and Written Directions

Verbal and written directions can be beneficial, in addition to observational learning, or by themselves. Clarity and simplicity are important considerations. Yet, there are many questions that need to be resolved with regard to instructional-directional techniques.

How much time should be allotted for free, uncontrolled participation in an activity? How much instruction, guidance, and demonstration is necessary, and at what point in the learning process are these teaching methods most beneficial?

Verbal encouragement and advice can no doubt assist the learner in mastering motor skills. However, personal experience and research (for example, Renshaw and Postle, 1928) suggest that on occasion too much direction offered by the teacher can hinder the learning of motor tasks. In this particular experiment, three groups of subjects were formed to learn to master the pursuit rotor task. Group I received a brief demonstration and was left alone; Group II, the analytical group, had some verbal directions in addition to the demonstration; and Group III was presented with detailed instructions and facts about the operation and manipulation of the apparatus.

An examination of Figure 6–4 shows that Group III clearly performed the poorest of the three groups. The other two groups performed about the same, and both were considerably better than Group III. Too much information or excessive guidance was detrimental to motor performance.

Mechanical Principles

Instruction need not be directed toward the execution of a specific act only. Information can also be provided about rules or principles that are potentially generalizable across a number of related tasks and situations. In mathematics, instructional approaches include the teaching of rules or principles that should help students solve problems in which such processes are applicable. The same reasoning can be applied to the teaching of motor skills.

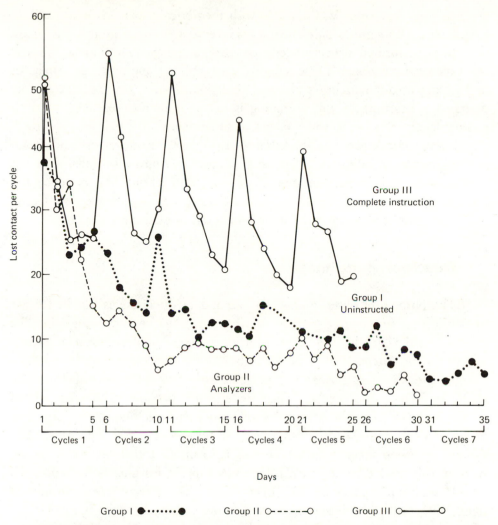

Figure 6–4. Group comparisons in motor performance under different types of instruction. A lowered performance curve indicates better performance. (From S. Renshaw and D. K. Postle, "Pursuit Learning Under Three Types of Instruction," *Journal of General Psychology,* 1, 1928, 360–367.)

Principles of movement, biochemical principles, can be taught to learners in order to facilitate the acquisition of skills learned later on. As is the case with any information related to skills learning, the effectiveness of this approach depends on the person's ability to understand and to use it.

One of the earliest studies (and perhaps most convincing) on the transference of a principle to the learning of a motor activity was reported by C. H. Judd in 1908. The task involved was tossing a dart at an underwater target. One group of subjects received no theoretical training but merely practiced, whereas the other group was provided with theoretical explanations in addition to practice. Although no difference in achievement between groups was found when they performed in twelve inches of water, a change to four inches favored the experimental group. These subjects were able to apply the principles of dart-tossing at different levels of water. Judd proposed a *generalization theory of transfer*. Learning by understanding is better than rote learning, for it is potentially transferable to wider ranges of situations.

Subsequent research on the learning of principles of movement and action on the learning of motor skills has led to somewhat equivocal results, although it does show some trends in support of such instruction. The evidence has been much stronger in the verbal learning area, where principles, strategies, and rules have been noted to be quite influential in classroom learnings.

Developing an Image

The purpose of observational learning and/or directions is for the learner to develop an internalized picture of what needs to be done—and then be able to do it. To "get the idea" implies the formation of an *internalized representation* of the act intended to be performed.

People who can visualize or "image" clearly tend to perform better. The ability to form an appropriate image depends on previous experience related to the learning task, the knowledge of appropriate techniques to form and strengthen the image, and concentration. In numerous verbal learning studies, various age-group subjects have been taught to improve their ability to image. In turn, this has led to improved achievement in the learning task studied.

In addition, John Shea (1977) has shown that *relevant labeling* results in significantly higher recall scores on a simple motor task. Labeling is a technique where the learner gives verbal cues to himself or herself, to make the learning experience more meaningful. It has been suggested by others that imagery is more effective when verbal tags are applied to and stored with the image. It would seem reasonable that the learner should attempt to image the act to be performed and attach to it appropriate verbal tags that are personally meaningful and relevant.

GOAL SETTING

Along with offering instructions to learners so that they become aware of the activity to be learned and what they need to do, it may be necessary to consider their performance goals. What is each person's expectations of herself or himself during the first practice session? Later? At the end of the unit? Are the goals too high? Too low? Indeed, are there any goals?

Within the context of motivational theory, and even practical wisdom, it is realized that the setting of meaningful short-term and long-term goals is extremely important. The word "meaningful" implies that goals should be realistic, related to present skill level and capabilities. Commitment to practice should be considered as well. More specific goals are easier to shoot for, and performance can be evaluated more precisely according to such goals. Furthermore, the goals should be high, but possible to attain. In other words, *goals should be specific, high, but attainable.*

A recent study by Mary Barnett and Jean Stanicek (1979) on the effects of goal setting in archery confirms the value of goals. Subjects in the goal-setting group were directed continuously to set numerical and verbal goals. The other group (control) did not receive such instructions. The goal-setting group achieved higher scores than the control group when they were tested. The establishment of specific goals is a valuable motivational technique.

Performance expectations should be established for each practice attempt, each session, throughout the entire program. They serve to motivate, they influence skill attainment, and they represent subordinate goals for the final goal.

The goals can and should be evaluated regularly and modified, upward or downward, when appropriate. After all, the goals may have been unrealistic. Or training may have been more or less effective and dedication to practice greater or lesser than expected.

Many students, through other experiences, may have learned how to establish performance goals. But most of them probably have not. The teacher's role is to assist learners with this process and procedure. Ideally, students will learn how to set realistic goals for themselves. Goals are based on previous successes and failures (as perceived by the learner) in the activity. For most individuals, success leads to higher performance expectations; failure leads to lower ones. Consequently, self-comparisons in performance may be more valuable on many occasions than comparison against others or against norms.

The establishment of hard but reachable goals is even more effective in influencing performance than trying to do one's best. This is nicely documented by Locke and Bryan in Figure 6–5. The subjects with specific and high goals did better on a motor task than those who were told to do their best. It can be seen that general or haphazard motivational techniques are not as effective as a precise technique such as goal setting.

The study of goal setting is not really new. In earlier years, it was referred to as *level of aspiration* in the literature. Now it is popularly termed *expectancy level* in motivational theory. To summarize, not only does appropriate goal setting induce greater performance, but levels of interest and motivation are enhanced

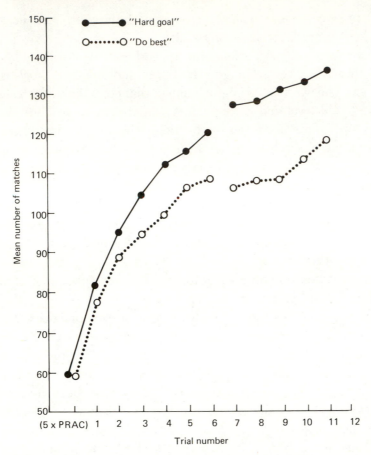

Figure 6–5. A comparison of two groups in performance on a complex motor task. One group had high standards and a difficult goal, the other group was merely told, "Do your best." The Hard-Goal group was significantly better than the Do-Best group. (From E. A. Locke, and J. F. Bryan, "Cognitive aspects of psychomotor performance: The effects of performance goals on level of performance," *Journal of Applied Psychology*, 50, 1966, 286–291.

also. And by the way, with the discussions on imagery and goal-setting, you are probably beginning to realize more and more how thought processes can influence feeling processes, and in turn motor learning/performance.

MODIFYING THE ACTIVITY AND LEARNING SITUATION

When possible, activities should be taught and learned as they will need to be performed. However, often motor skills are so complex to the learner that some modification in the learning environment or teaching method may have to be made. Teaching methods, and alternatives, will be discussed shortly. For now, let's focus on the task and its environment. More specifically, the nature of cues, trainers, and simulators will be addressed.

A person can only handle so much information at one time. Consequently, the practice situation should encourage concentration on the most relevant cue(s) at any point prior to and during the execution of an act or activity. Cues can be given verbally, such as the ever-famous "keep your eye on the ball." Verbal cues and prompts prior to and during an activity may help the learner to single out the most important information to attend to, thereby making it easier for him or her to learn/perform.

But "visual" cues may serve their purpose, too. For instance, in reaction time studies, a warning signal (light or noise) usually results in a faster reaction time. Visual cues in the form of dots or arrows when the bowler is supposed to release the ball are easier to focus on than the pins at the end of the alley. At times it may be advantageous to add visual cues in the situation that are not normally found in it. They may help learners learn to focus at appropriate places during performance. A word of caution is in order, though. As a general rule, supplementary cues *should be removed as soon as possible.* Learners should not learn to depend on cues that will not be available in the "real" situation.

The same principle is true when any type of artifical aid is added to the learning environment, as with trainers. *Trainers* are usually constructed pieces of equipment that reduce the overall complexity of the demands of the task on the student. We see them used in all types of sports. For example, ball-tossing machines aid tennis players and baseball players as balls are delivered in a predictable fashion. This allows learners to concentrate on the mechanics of the movement. They need not be concerned with uncertainties of ball speed and placement. When trainers are used, the objective is to derive value from them and then progress the student to the next level of performance. Perhaps more advanced trainers will be used. But as soon as possible they should be removed so that learners can develop all of the skills necessary to perform under real performance conditions.

Simulators, on the other hand, are usually devices that more nearly approximate real conditions. Although fake cockpits and automobile controls have been devised for simulating practice flying an airplane or driving a car, most athletic skills do not require the usage of such costly and complex equipment. Yet golf can be learned in the gymnasium with the use of plastic or taped balls. Simulated skiing conditions have been constructed to aid people to learn to ski in the absence of snow. The more devices approximate real conditions, the better the learner can acquire and maintain skills in the absence of "the real thing."

Mechanical or equipment aids acting as simulators or trainers have been found to be beneficial in a number of circumstances. In some instances, this has not been the case. In yet others, conflicting research findings pose a dilemma for the potential user of a particular trainer or simulator. Let us examine a case in point.

The Golfer's Groove is a mechanical device that guides the golfer's swing. It guides the learner's club along a theoretically correct plane while he or she generates the required level of force. Some evidence was reported in the literature to support its use in the instruction of beginners. However, with greater experimental controls, Gary Skrinar and Shirl Hoffman (1978) did not note any advantage in the use of this "aid." Skill test scores and swing ratings were not any different between a group using the Golfer's Groove and one not using it. In a situation where conflicting evidence is reported with regard to the use of a particular apparatus, one has to evalaute the procedures in the studies carefully to determine weaknesses and strengths. If the procedures that led to conflicting results are somewhat similar in the control of potential biases or artifacts, then further evidence is needed to resolve the issue.

WHOLE VERSUS PART PRACTICE

Modifications in practice situations need not involve only physical rearrangement, special cues, trainers, and simulators. The activity itself can be simplified in how it is practiced. In other words, the practice of a task can proceed in its entirety, or else it can be fractionated into sub-units or parts. Thus, alternatives are available: to practice a skill by the *whole* method or the *part* method.

Many activities can be broken down into parts for purposes of instruction, or taught in their entirety. Take the crawl stroke in swimming, for example. One could teach the leg kick, arm stroke, and breathing separately or together. The golf swing could be separated into sequential parts and taught that way, or taught as a "whole." As a general rule, simple activities indicate the whole method, while difficult activities require the part method first, the whole method later.

But how do we define what is simple and what is complex to learn? Sometimes the answer is simple, at other times not. The conceptual orientation of psychologists James Naylor and George Briggs (1963) helps us to analyze motor tasks against meaningful criteria in order to make decisions about practice.

The two major criteria, task complexity and task organization, are suggested, where *task complexity* is a function of the information processing and memory demands placed on the learner, and *task organization* refers to the nature of relationship of its components.

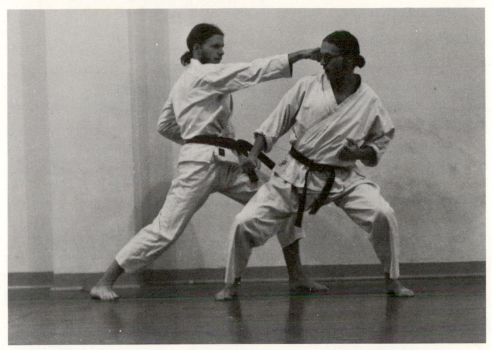

Featherkill Studios, Burnsville, MN

One consideration in using the part practice technique in learning an activity is the danger to the participants.

To go into more detail, task complexity considers the kinds and amounts of perceptions and information needed to be attended to, and how difficult it is to remember to what and how to respond. Task organization considers the kinds of movements to be made, their timing and sequence. A highly organized task is one in which the bodily parts may be synchronized in action. There may be few movements. The low-organized task is just the opposite.

For example, the crawl swimming stroke probably contains moderate task complexity but rather low organization. The organization is low because although the leg kick is synchronized, it's an action quite different from the arm pattern. Then there is the breathing pattern to consider. Most swimming instructors would probably teach the crawl with the part method at first.

Golf instructors differ in opinion as to how to teach the golf stroke. The stroke seems to possess moderate task complexity and organization. The stroke can be broken down into progressive parts such as readiness stance, partial back-stroke, completed backstroke, partial follow-through (where ball contact would be), and completed follow-through. Depending on the feelings of the teacher and the abilities of the learner, the stroke could be learned in its entirety or in parts.

Wherever possible, the whole method is more desirable as it saves time. But the refined learning of the mechanics of a movement, especially one that requires a number of subroutines, suggests practice on the parts until they are learned well enough to be put together as a whole movement unit, and performed as if automatically.

An interesting perspective to the whole/part training question has been addressed by Mary Jo Murray (1979). She considered two possible meaningful ways individuals might differ as to their preferred cognitive approach to learning. Subjects, on the basis of an inventory test, were classified as either holistic or sequential information processors. They had to learn a juggling task. Murray found that the sequential learners using the part method and the holistic learners using the whole method took fewer minutes to learn the activity than did the sequential learners using the whole method and the holistic learners using the part method. This study emphasized the point made throughout this book: appropriate teaching and learning techniques are those that reflect careful task analysis and person analysis.

MENTAL PRACTICE

Earlier in this chapter we talked about imagery, or getting the idea of what was to be performed. Imagery is the ability to construct an internalized mental picture of the intended act. *Mental practice* is an extension of this activity. It includes not only forming an image, but repeatedly mentally rehearsing it.

The value of mental practice (also called *mental rehearsal* or *covert rehearsal*) has been verified in research as well as by the statements of many outstanding athletes. In the latter case, numerous athletes have reported mentally rehearsing their skills and imaging contest-like conditions the night before or the morning before a contest. One might argue that this activity helps to strengthen performance, since mental activity activates nerve impulses and the corresponding parts of the body. In a way, it also serves as a self pre-cuing technique. It may enhance motivation.

Research in this area is not new. The classic experimental paradigm is to form two groups of subjects, one of which will not mentally rehearse a novel motor task, one of which will do so. Invariably, the mentally-practiced group does better that the control group when physically attempting to perform the task. In some research, a third group is formed: a physical practice group that

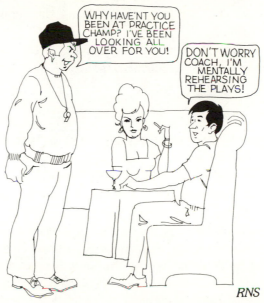

From Singer, R. N.: Myths and Truths in Sports Psychology. *New York: Harper & Row, 1975.*

practices the task as often as the mental practice group. As might be expected, this group will achieve higher than the other two groups. In other studies, a fourth group has been designated, one that receives a combination of mental and physical practice. This group will probably perform as well or slightly less well than a physical practice group.

In a typical experiment, Charles Corbin (1967) formed three groups to determine the value of mental rehearsal in the learning of a motor task: a wand-juggling task. All subjects actually practiced the task for five consecutive days. Afterwards, the mental practice and the physical practice groups practiced the task 30 times daily for 13 days. The control group received no additional practice. On subsequent tests, the control group did not improve, and were not expected to. Also as expected, the physical practice group was superior. However, mental practice did seem to facilitate actual skill acquisition.

It can be seen that the best motor learning occurs with overt (physical) practice. Mental practice, however, is more effective than no practice at all. Highly skilled athletes have adopted their own particular practice strategies in terms of the use of mental rehearsal (when, how often, how long). Usually this is not done in the formalized manner administered in research settings.

Even in experiments, mental rehearsal techniques vary. One typical approach is to give instructions, verbal or visual, and have subjects rehearse the act a certain number of times. Subjects are requested to think through the act in detail. They are asked to see themselves making the appropriate movement in the specified situation.

In the athletic world, more and more sport psychologists are designing psychological training programs to enhance athletes' abilities to relax, concentrate, image, and mentally practice.

MENTALLY PRACTICING AN ACTIVITY

Why don't you try your hand (or shall we say your mind) at mentally rehearsing a motor act? Let's take something familar to all of us, the foul shot (free throw) in basketball.

First of all, relax. Close your eyes. Be comfortable in your chair. Envision standing at the foul line with a basketball in your hand. Now see the rim. Study it. Be relaxed at the foul line, bounce the ball a few times, concentrate on the rim of the basket, and shoot the ball when ready. See the ball go into the basket. When ready, repeat the act. Do it ten times.

Were you able to see yourself in the act? What details, if any, stood out? Could you imagine the ball going in the basket? If it missed, you're in trouble!

Did you find parts of your body moving (without any deliberate intention on your part) as you imagined the act? This is a fairly common occurrence if you're really into the mental rehearsal process.

SPEED AND ACCURACY

As we all realize, there is optimal quickness and accuracy for each kind of activity. Assuming that both factors may be equally important in skilled performance, should an act be practiced in a slowed-down manner, with emphasis on the movement and form? Should speed in movement be emphasized, reasoning that accuracy will come later? Or should both speed and precision be emphasized equally in learning?

The usual approach is to stress movement form and accuracy, gradually increasing the speed of execution as practice proceeds. Yet, it might be detrimental to do this. Let's look to tennis for an example. A child could learn a tennis skill with very nice form, yet hit the ball very gently. But under competitive conditions, he or she eventually will have to hit firmer and harder. The movement must be quickened. Essentially, different combinations of muscle fibers and motor units need to be innervated (activated) as to timing and force application.

Although it is usually more frustrating at first to practice a skill under both speed and accuracy conditions, this may be the best approach in the long run. Watch beginners play. They merely want to get the ball over the net, into the court. They push at the ball. They'll do anything to get the ball over, to gain some sense of self-perceived satisfaction. As has been known so long (and quantified by the late Paul Fitts and ultimately called Fitts' Law), a definite and predictable relationship exists between the speed and accuracy of a movement on one hand and the target's size and its distance from the person on the other.

That is, with speed we lose accuracy and with accuracy we lose speed. When targets are larger and closer to us, fewer detrimental effects are seen when we attempt to move quickly and accurately to a target. In the tennis example, although accuracy in stroking was gained initially, it was, in a sense, attained under "false" conditions. As was stated before, later the stroke must be modified to produce a harder (and still accurate) hit. Probably if the learner had started out by stroking firmly, the best ultimate results would have been realized.

The general rule is that *practice conditions should resemble contest (or later expected) conditions as much as possible.*

There are exceptions to this rule, of course. First, the nature of certain tasks, in terms of complexity or danger, may require initial modifications in the way they are practiced. Second, a student who has difficulty in improving may need extra attention and special modified practice conditions. Perhaps the movement should be slowed down so that special problems can be worked out. We certainly want to minimize frustration and lack of reasonable progress.

SPEED VERSUS ACCURACY EFFECTS ON LEARNING A TENNIS STROKE

It is true that some research findings support the notion of gradually working up to the speed demands of a task—starting at lesser speed and increasing it. However, the principle of equal instructional emphasis on speed and accuracy simultaneously is a good one to remember in most situations. Physical educator John Woods illustrated this point very nicely in an article appearing in a 1967 issue of the *Research Quarterly.* The forehand tennis stroke was the skill to be learned. Three groups of subjects were formed, and they practiced for five weeks.

Group I practiced under maximum ball velocity conditions for 12 days and then under maximum ball-placement accuracy conditions for 12 days. Group II practiced under the reverse conditions. Group III concentrated on an equal and simultaneous attainment of velocity and accuracy for the entire 24 days of instruction and practice. Then all three groups were tested as to ball velocity and accuracy when stroking. Woods concluded that for a skill that requires equal emphasis on both ball velocity and placement accuracy (in this case, the tennis forehand stroke) the most desirable results are obtained by equal and simultaneous practice on both variables.

PROBLEM-SOLVING VERSUS GUIDED LEARNING

A teacher can attempt to structure the learning experience so that students are guided and prompted continually. Thinking (improvising, planning, adaptive) behaviors would be discouraged. Learning is efficient, as specific acts are acquired quickly. This approach is called *guided learning.*

Alternatively, students can attempt to acquire skills spontaneously in a trial and error manner, under discovery or problem-solving procedures. These in turn can be completely free (the learners are not guided at all) or guided—tactfully—by the instructor. This is termed *problem-solving learning;* it takes more time but increases the probability of adapting to new but related situations. In terms of instructional decisions, much depends on the preferred techniques of the teacher and the intended outcomes of the learning situation.

If what is desired is the most *efficient and effective means* of acquiring a skill or skills, then highly guided learning techniques would be preferable. If the purpose of the learning situation is to lead to the development of the *learning process,* to get learners to think, resolve any situational dilemmas, adapt, and transfer old learnings to new but related situations, then the encouragement of problem-solving approaches in the initial learning settings should be advantageous. Remember our discussion of open (externally-paced) and closed (self-paced) tasks earlier in the book? Closed tasks require repetitious practice, and the development of habit-like acts. Open tasks involve adaptive processes, the ability to react suddenly to the unknown, and anticipation. Habit-like learned acts could be disastrous to performance in open situations. When you are in control of the ball in a basketball game, you have to deal with each situation in the appropriate manner. Rigid habits may cause you to make mistakes.

As can be seen in Figure 6–6, differences in learning and performance occur in trial and error (discovery) conditions and error-free (highly cued) conditions. Subjects had to learn a serial manipulation task, one that required hand

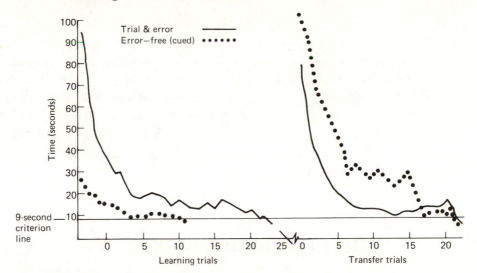

Figure 6–6. A comparison of the effectiveness of cued learning and trial-and-error learning on acquisition and transfer. (From R. N. Singer and L. Gaines, "Effects of prompted and problem-solving approaches on learning and transfer of motor skills," *American Educational Research Journal,* 12, 1975, 395–404.)

movements to correct objects in the right sequence and as quickly as possible. There are two obvious conclusions:

(1) the learning of a task without any prior experience is favored under heavily prompted and cued conditions.
(2) the learning of a second and related task (transfer) is favored after the first task has been learned under problem-solving conditions.

Long-term benefits in achievement will be obtained by practice in varied situations, encouraging the learner to think, understand, and be prepared for eventualities. Adaptability to situations can only occur with practices that encourage problem-solving and flexibility in behaviors. Robot-like learnings are ineffective in open tasks. A switching mechanism needs to be developed, from automatic behaviors to adjustive behaviors.

Therefore, the issue of guided learning versus problem-solving learning is not really an issue but rather a decision to be made depending on the nature of the activity and intended goals. Both techniques are effective. But each serves a different purpose.

Structured practice—drill—is highly effective with closed tasks. Grooving movements, like those in golf and archery, will benefit from repetitious practice.

In activities that might require adjustive behaviors, students need the opportunity to practice under varied conditions so as to be prepared for the unexpected.

Guided learning is highly efficient, leading to specifically acquired behavior. Problem-solving learning takes more time but increases the probability of adapting to new but related situations. Many practice sessions may include both types of approaches. A careful analysis of the activities you are teaching and the current and potential future demands on the student will help you decide on how much emphasis should be placed on guided *(product)* learning versus problem-solving *(process)* learning.

THE DISTRIBUTION OF PRACTICE

There is only so much time to practice, and yet there are so many skills we hope that students will learn well in an activity program. A question often raised is, how much continuous *(massed)* practice should be allotted to the perfecting of a particular skill in an instructional unit? Should practice in that skill be broken up frequently by rest periods or by practice in other skills *(distributed)?*

Continuous practice is undesirable with:

(1) younger children, because their attention span is relatively brief and tends to wander.
(2) adult beginners, for they usually have the same problem.
(3) fatiguing tasks, as incorrect behavioral patterns will be practiced by tired students.
(4) dangerous tasks, because someone might get hurt if fatigue occurs.

With more highly skilled and conditioned performers, massed practice is accepted more readily and can be effective. A general summary of the extensive research literature on the topic of the effectiveness of massed versus distributed practice, across a wide range of skills, indicates that immediate performance is more effective under distributed practice. In the few studies in which long-term retention has been studied, usually no differences in achievement level is observed. The massed practice subjects seem to improve while the distributed practice subjects worsen, and eventually both hit the same level.

In other words, massed practice on occasion results in a temporary dip in performance. Learning is occurring, but performance worsens due to boredom or fatigue. A phenomenon called *reminiscence* is observed. Reminiscence is im-

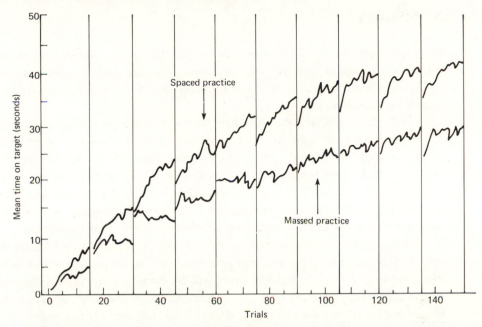

Figure 6–7. Learning curves for massed and distributed practice groups. Within each block of 20 trials, the distributed practice group rested between trials while the massed practice group performed continuously. Following a rest after each 20 trials for each group, the distributed practice demonstrates early decrements from preceding performance, the massed group shows early increments, but the distributed group remains constantly superior to the massed group. Note the similar patterns within each group within each block of 20 trials. (From G. A. Kimble and R. B. Shatel, The Relationship between two kinds of inhibition and the amount of practice, *Journal of Experimental Psychology,* 1952, 44, 355–359.)

provement in performance over time, during a period of no practice. It's as if too much continuous practice is a temporary damper on achievement. With time, such inhibitory processes disappear, and a truer skill level is demonstrated.

To mass or distribute practice of a specific skill, therefore, may not make too much of a difference in the long run, as far as achievement is concerned. However, most educators favor some form or degree of distribution of practice for motivational and other purposes.

A typical study in the area is presented in Figure 6–7. It can be observed that performance on the pursuit rotor apparatus resulted in higher performance under spaced practice than under massed practice. These findings are commonplace across a variety of learning materials. It should be noted that in those studies in which the long-range effects (retention) of such practice schedules have been investigated, very little difference is found when comparing group performances at a later date.

SUMMARY

Practice conditions should be favorable as possible as the quickest means to establish the highest level of skill, considering the way learners can react to guidance procedures and situations. There is no reason why learning experiences cannot be enjoyable, too.

Well-planned, systematic procedures lead to a higher probability of successful instructional outcomes. In this perspective, systems models of instruction were described, indicating the nature of such an approach. The science of instruction relies heavily on research on the psychology of learning and applications of it that can be derived. Teachers need to teach learners how to acquire appropriate learning strategies, both techniques of value to motor tasks in general and task-specific skills. Consequently, many possibilities need to be considered.

When learning a motor skill, conditions and strategies can be identified prior to practice, during practice, and after practice. Certain considerations were identified in this chapter. Related topics will be discussed in the next chapter. At the start of any learning unit, the student must "get the idea" of what is to be accomplished. An activity is introduced to the learner. Various techniques, alone or in combination, can be used to achieve this purpose. Observational learning—the modeling effect—is very effective. Verbal and/or written directions, with or without viewing the intended performance, can also be an effective means of transmitting information. Whatever the technique, the information processing capacities and capabilities of the learners must be considered, to determine the amount of information to be used and be useful at one time. Obviously, the quality of any technique used is important, too.

Mechanical principles should lead to a better understanding of what to do (and why to do it) in the present situation, as well as in future related circumstances. Whatever techniques are communicated by the teacher, the learner needs to be able to internalize this information. The internalization process is associated with the creation of a mental image, an image of the intended act. Along with this image goes the formation of goals. Goals, or performance expectations, are related to past perceived successes and failures in similar situations. Most meaningful performance goals are those that are specifically defined, high, but attainable.

As to actual practice, the task or environment can be modified at first to accommodate the learner. Cuing, aiding, and simulating procedures can be quite effective with beginners attempting to master difficult tasks. They can reduce stimulus uncertainty and movement complexity. But they should be removed gradually and eliminated as soon as possible. Tasks can be broken down into parts or learned as "wholes." Applying criteria of task organization and task difficulty, decisions can be made as to the desirability of the part versus whole practice method. The best practice is that which occurs under "real" conditions. Such practice prepares the person for what needs to be done under what circumstances, when he or she confronts performance conditions that have not been modified artificially for learning purposes.

Mental practice, an extension of imagery, has been demonstrated to be an effective learning or performance maintenance technique. As to speed and accuracy in the practice of movements, the tradeoff is obvious: emphasis on one diminishes the effectiveness of the other. Task analysis is necessary. Emphasis on either speed or accuracy or both should usually be reflected by how the task is ultimately to be performed. Another issue is whether to guide the learning of an activity with many prompts or cues, or to allow students to problem-solve and discover appropriate behaviors in particular situations. Formal guidance is highly efficient for the acquisition of specific skills or knowledges. Problem-solving situations take more time but may be more effective in aiding retention and promoting transfer possibilities (learning related skills).

In this chapter we have addressed the establishment of favorable practice conditions for learners in general. But it would be helpful to understand the learning processes we are attempting to influence. Obviously, the ultimate intention is to improve the mechanics of particular movements and the application of strategies in order to achieve reasonable performance goals. In the next chapter, we will consider some of the more important learning processes involved in the possible realization of such goals. Inferences will also be drawn as to what constitutes improved practice conditions that enhance the operation of these processes.

REFERENCES AND SUGGESTED READINGS

Barnett, M. L. and Stanicek, J. A. Effects of goal setting on achievement in archery. *Research Quarterly,* 1979, 50, 328–332.

Corbin, C. B. Effects of mental practice on skill development after controlled practice. *Research Quarterly,* 1967, 38, 534–538.

Glaser, R. Components of a psychology of instruction: toward a science of design. *Review of Educational Research,* 1976, 46, 1–24.

Joyce, B. and Weil, M. *Models of teaching,* second edition. Englewood Cliffs, N.J.: Prentice-Hall, 1980.

Locke, E. A. and Bryan, J. F. Cognitive aspects of psychomotor performance: the effects of performance goals on level of performance. *Journal of Applied Psychology,* 1966, 50, 286–291.

Murray, M. J. Matching preferred cognitive mode with teaching methodology in learning a novel motor skill. *Research Quarterly,* 1979, 50, 80–87.

Naylor, J. C. and Briggs, G. E. Long-term retention of learned skills: a review of the literature. *ASD Technical Report 61–390,* U.S. Department of Commerce, 1963.

Shea, J. B. Effects of labelling on motor short-term memory. *Journal of Experimental Psychology,* 1977, 3, 92–99.

Singer, R. N. *Motor learning and human performance,* third edition. New York: Macmillan Publishing Co., Inc. 1980, Chapters 11, 12, and 13.

Singer, R. N. The learning system approach an instruction in psychomotor activities. *Motor Skills: Theory into Practice,* 1977, 1, 113–122.

Singer, R. N. To err or not to err: A question for the instruction of psychomotor skills. *Review of Educational Research,* 1977, 47, 479–498.

Singer, R. N. and Dick, W. *Teaching physical education: a systems approach.* Boston: Houghton Mifflin, 1980.

Skrinar, G. S. and Hoffman, S. J. Mechanical guidance of the golf swing: the golfer's groove as an instructional adjunct. *Research Quarterly,* 1978, 49, 335–341.

Thomas, J. R., Pierce, C., and Ridsdale, S. Age differences in children's ability to model motor behavior. *Research Quarterly,* 1977, 48, 592–597.

Woods, J. B. The effect of varied instructional emphasis upon the development of a motor skill. *Research Quarterly,* 1967, 38, 132–141.

7

LEARNER
PROCESSES

Generally speaking, regardless of person and skill level, a series of internal processes are activated from the time learning/performance begins until an act or sequence of acts is completed. These processes are controlled differently by different people. People's capacities function to the degree that they are used efficiently and appropriately. Thus, although countless factors influence achievement in motor skills, one factor has to do with when and how internal processes are activated and controlled.

In this chapter we will address topics that deal with the learner's psychological processes that are associated with the ability to learn and achieve at motor skills. Readiness state, selective attention, attentional focus, anticipation, arousal level, memory, decision-making, and information feedback are associated with the achievement of most skills. An understanding of how these processes operate should suggest ways to influence them so that they function appropriately. These processes will then be incorporated in a proposed model of motor behavior.

Skilled athletes are skilled for a number of reasons, one of which is their ability to use their psychological capacities to fullest advantage. Abilities associated with processes that every learner/performer activates, consciously or not, are:

(1) to prepare oneself to be in the best state to learn or perform.
(2) to selectively attend to the most important cues or information in a situation.
(3) to concentrate.
(4) to anticipate potential immediate events (as in an externally-paced task).
(5) to sustain an optimal arousal (emotional) level.

133

(6) to use memory and contribute to it as appropriate.

(7) to make decisions effectively (prior to or during an act, depending on circumstances, with regard to execution).

(8) to use pertinent feedback information after and possibly during performance when desirable. The degree of conscious (deliberate) level of control over these depends on skill level, experiences, and what is most advantageous. When we analyze characteristics of highly skilled performers in Chapter 9, the way internal processes operate, indeed should operate, will take on added significance. In the meanwhile, we turn to a very important and well recognized factor in one's ability to learn to perform a motor task.

STATE OF READINESS

Readiness to learn and perform can be interpreted as the student's willingness, receptivity, or desire to acquire information and skills, and in general to perform well. We will not consider maturational or developmental readiness here. These areas were considered earlier in the book.

Several factors may influence a person's psychological preparatory state:

(1) prior experience, familiarity, and skill level in the present activity.

(2) previous successes in the same or similar activities.

(3) cognitive style (personal approaches to addressing and solving problems).

(4) attitudes and feelings toward and in the situation.

Students, athletes, or any performers must be psychologically and physically ready to learn if, indeed, they are going to learn. They must be ready to perform (as in athletic contests or dance renditions) if they are going to perform well. They need to be able to identify dispositional states to learn/perform by self-evaluation techniques. Self-analysis training, with an understanding of what to do about particular problems, should therefore facilitate the effectiveness of students in a variety of circumstances.

As is the case with the learning or performance of specific skills, learning how to be prepared, oriented, or ready to perform motor skills is a major factor in the determination of performance outcomes. Optimal attitudinal and arousal states for each task and each person should be determined. Arousal (emotions) relative to skill achievement will be covered shortly. It suffices to suggest here that learners need the ability to channel their motivation and emotions so that the ideal arousal and attentional condition is exhibited for the task to be learned (Landers, 1980). Closely related factors associated with both thoughts and feelings influence the learning of motor skills. More successful learners and performers have learned how to control and direct these thoughts and emotional processes appropriately for a particular activity and situation. This is true, of course, not only prior to performance, but during and after as well.

INFORMATION PROCESSING CAPABILITIES

A model of motor behavior will be proposed briefly in a little while. A series of internal processes and mechanisms activated during the performance of a motor act will be discussed.

From a simplified perspective, we must realize that a number of processes operate during the learning/performance of an activity, mainly:

(1) receiving information, cues, signals.
(2) making sense of it (or them).
(3) decision making as to what to do.
(4) responding (or withholding a response).
(5) using feedback (when appropriate).

In the information-processing perspective, information is transformed as it is passed along the system. It is *encoded*, that is, transformed into a general form to be stored in the system. And, there are times that it is *decoded*—transformed from the more abstract form to a less abstract form, to facilitate retrieval and decision-making processes. The way and the extent to which transformations are made on information affect the speed and accuracy of the processing. This is one of the major reasons why some learners are more effective than others. The more successful students have learned how to process information more efficiently and thus more effectively.

It is one thing to understand the mechanics of a movement; it is something else to be ready to practice and learn them. The more expediently and correctly information can be received and processed in the system, the more likely it is that the movement behavior will be the appropriate one. Obviously, psychological, biomechanical, and physiological processes interact and contribute to meaningful and purposeful execution, or skill.

The learning of any athletic skill requires attention to appropriate cues at any given time, the ability to interpret the present events in terms of previous experience, and decision-making, which calls for the execution of the correct response timed appropriately to the situational demands. During actual competitive performance, acquired skills need to be expressed under varying conditions of personal control, from deliberate conscious intervention to what appears as automatic or semi-automatic response. In other words, "Proficiency is determined by the capability to achieve predetermined goals, either through an automatic run of a program or with the modification of behavior through effective use of internalized feedback to adapt to unpredicted or unusual circumstances" (Singer, 1978, p. 102).

By understanding those processes that the human uses from the point information is received until performance occurs (and after it occurs) one can attempt to determine ways of facilitating the operation of them. Various processes help to control and therefore determine the ultimate quality of motor behavior as a result of the way information is received, managed, and directed. Thus, individual variations in the operation of perceptual, attentional, memorial, decisional, and motor mechanisms help to contribute to the ultimate skill level that is evidenced by different persons. More specifically, the manner in which a learner utilizes various processes in relation to personal capabilities is one of the major determinants of individual differences in the acquisition of skill. Good learner abilities in this regard help to contribute to higher degrees of learning and performance.

Let us examine the human system, and the flow of events from the time a person receives information (a cue) until a response (the behavior) is actually made. The operant subsystems seem to operate in a sequential (sometime parallel) way as illustrated in Figure 7–1. From a learning point of view, we would want to know how to improve upon those processes associated with the boxes that appear in that illustration. A review of Chapter 2, and familiarity with concepts from information processing, cybernetic, and hierarchical control models, would provide helpful background information.

RECEIVING, USING, AND PROCESSING SENSORY INFORMATION

The learner must learn what information, signals, or cues are pertinent to respond to in a particular circumstance. *The senses*, each with unique functions, are the means by which we take in information, which is stored temporarily in

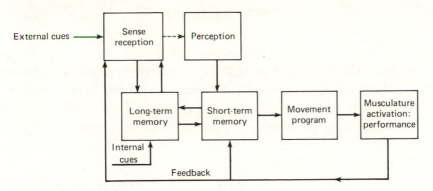

FIGURE 7–1. The flow of information from various input sources to performance. A complex series of operations occurs to transform information and expectations to meaningful movement behavior. (From R. N. Singer and W. Dick. *Teaching Physical Education: A Systems Approach,* 2nd ed. Boston: Houghton Mifflin, 1980.)

the senses before being processed by higher centers in the nervous system. A greater amount of information is never "recognized" internally; it is never really processed further. This is because stimuli have to be of sufficient magnitude or they won't trigger additional internal processing. Most of the stimuli that surround us, however, are not of such magnitude.

This is why learners need to identify the *minimal, most relevant cues* in a performance situation. They must *selectively attend* to cues, since only a limited amount of information can be attended to or processed at one time. An additional but important consideration in receiving information is the *functional state* of those sense receptors associated with achievement in a particular activity.

For many years the wrong children were identified in the classroom as being slow learners or mentally retarded. They were "wrong" in the sense that these children were found to have sensory handicaps, such as with vision or hearing, rather than with their intelligence. In other words, an inability to receive the correct information hampered their learning and achievement in the classroom. When corrective devices were used or teaching modified to take sensory limitations into considerations, these same students could achieve according to standard expectations. In sports, vision is extremely important where ball detection has to occur quickly or playing situations have to be scanned in a brief period of time. Hearing the teacher's cues or instructions is also important in many sports activities. Many examples can be offered. Can you think of others? The important thing here is consideration of the functional state of senses, so that the human system takes in appropriate information in its true form and at the right time.

PERCEPTION

Once information is forwarded within the nervous system, it has to be given some *meaning*. The process of perception is associated with making meaning; stimuli are detected and recognized. Information that has been stored in the long-term memory from previous similar experiences help the functioning of the perceptual process. Obviously, relevant previous learnings, and the ability to retrieve such helpful information, both enhance overall performance capabilities in the present situation.

Once meaning has been attached to stimuli, further appropriate processing can occur. In a truly unfamiliar situation, responses are delayed considerably, as information processing takes much longer. Of course, until perceptions are right, responses do not have a high probability of being adequate. Perceptions are also enhanced when the process of attention is working favorably. Attention in this sense may be associated with cue selection, concentration, and arousal level within a person.

ATTENTION

Attention refers to an individual's *readiness* in a particular situation to *selectively* receive and process information. Attention is associated with many aspects of information processing and performance, because attentional capabilities provide the framework for what we can do and how we do it. Likewise, the state of arousal may be considered in the same way. Similarities in the concepts of attention and arousal have been noted, as well as differences. A most important conclusion, however, in regard to both of them, is that *there is an optimal level of attention and arousal for each person and for each act.*

The challenge for the learner is to learn how to control and influence his or her own attentional and arousal states. The challenge for the instructor is to analyze each act and activity in terms of demands placed on the learner, then analyze each learner in terms of ability to control and direct attentional and emotional processes, and to help learners individually to develop abilities to cope with the learning situation.

We will return to the notion of arousal state later in this chapter. Motivation, a related topic, will be dealt with in the next chapter. For now, a series of topics of interest related to attention will be covered.

Preparation of the Learner

Attention is integral to the learner's preparedness to learn. In one sense, attention or attentiveness can refer to the *readiness* of a person to receive certain information and process it. It is implied in this statement that a degree of motivation is present as well.

Anticipation

The importance of anticipating behavior in certain externally-paced activities cannot be emphasized enough. As a person becomes skilled, he or she needs to give less conscious attention to the immediate activity. More attention can be directed toward subsequent possibilities—possible maneuvers to be made against an opponent, or tactics an opponent may use.

We have a limited capacity to take in information and deal with it. Our mental system can be freed to anticipate more, and learners need to learn how, when, and to what to anticipate. Expecting what might happen, being prepared to react accordingly, and then executing correctly is the ideal sequence of events. There are times when it is better not to anticipate. But one of the major problems many athletes have is not thinking ahead to possible circumstances and what should be done in them. Reading cues quickly, such as judging where on your court the opposing tennis player is going to return the ball, allows you to be in the proper place in plenty of time to execute mechanically and initiate an offensive strategy.

Anticipation can also be examined in a more restricted sense than described so far. Even in an isolated act, the correct anticipation of the speed and placement of a projectile (for example, a ball) allows the athlete to be in the proper place to catch it or kick it, or to apply a piece of equipment (like a bat) to it. The process of anticipation leads to better *timing* of the response to the stimulus.

Concentration as Blockage of Interfering Thoughts

During a specific act, concentration on a specific object or thought not only enhances attention but will also help to *block out irrelevant thoughts*. It is common to think too much in an activity. In an act like hitting a baseball, shooting a free throw in basketball, or diving off the board, the athlete must learn to concentrate on a particular cue, so that the whole body "does its thing."

Trying to think during the act about parts of the body and where they are is counterproductive. So is worrying about execution. The time to think, if at all, is before the act. And thinking should be positive. In self-paced tasks like rolling a bowling ball, the person has time to put himself or herself in an

optimal relaxed state
   to be followed by
brief imagery (a mental picture of the intended act)
   to be followed by
attention to a specific cue (in bowling, the arrow on the alley)
   leading to
execution (doing it without any conscious attention to the act)

The same principle holds true for externally-paced tasks. The major difference is that there may not be time to preset oneself. The psychological processes mentioned above need to be speeded up. Attention to the ball—trying to see the seams of the ball—takes up attentional space. There is no "mental space," or capacity, to think of anything else.

Selective Situational Cues

Selective attention is the process by which a learner selects from all available sources of information that which will be attended to for the purposes of the particular activity. It should be apparent that the ability to selectively attend to information is an important requirement in any learning circumstance. And, because situations vary in predictable and unpredictable ways, selective-attention processes must be anticipatory, flexible, and adaptable, to accommodate changing information. This allows a person to monitor the most appropriate cues at any given time. Ideally, a person attends to the minimum number of cues that provide the maximum amount of information in any given situation.

The Maintenance of Attention

Some activities are very brief, like throwing a shot or swimming in a 100-meter event. Others, like basketball games or tennis matches, take some time to complete. Attentional level must be maintained throughout competition. Considering attention in this way allows us to deal with *concentration*. One of the more difficult attributes to develop, concentration—the maintenance of attention throughout the duration of an activity—can make the difference in achievement.

Mental lapses cause errors in performance. Many tennis players and golfers admit to problems in sustaining attention over time. This capability, like any other, be it primarily mechanical or psychological, must be trained. The continual contention here is that the mind and body should be considered *together* in practice or training programs. Therefore, *practice should simulate contest situations whenever possible.* Athletes must train hard, and not take practice for granted, in order to prepare adequately for competition. It is unfortunate that psychological processes are not trained more conscientiously in practice.

Capacity

People are like water hoses—fortunately, only in a very small way. Both have a *limited capacity:* the former to attend to and process information; the latter to circulate water.

A theoretical *filtering* mechanism is responsible for allowing appropriate cues into the human system while at the same time keeping out irrelevant ones. And in most cases only one cue can be consciously attended to at one time. When simultaneous information is presented to a person, some of it is put on temporary hold, and is responded to subsequently. The process occurs so fast that it may appear that we process much information simultaneously. There are exceptions that we will consider shortly, when we discuss single-channel and multi-channel models of attention.

Attention is associated with the various operations or stages that are activated sequentially, from the selection of a cue to which to respond, to the actual response. Indeed, Geoffrey Underwood (1978), recognizing the important role of attention in the way we function, refers to attention as a *control process.* Attention can (if we wish to become consciously involved) control what information is selected to be processed and what processes are used to be performed on this information, leading to decision-making as to what to do. With skill, many stages of processing may be performed without attention. The learning of when and how to use attention is associated with the process of becoming a skilled performer.

When we think of paying attention to something, the question that naturally arises is: How much attention can be allocated at one time to receive and process the pertinent information? What is our capacity? Can we do two things at one time? Only one thing at a time?

Alternative viewpoints have appeared in the literature. The *single channel model,* as proposed by Donald Broadbent in 1958 and slightly later by A. T.

Welford, is associated with the basic premise that we can only attend to one thing at a time. Information gets processed sequentially. Others believe that there is an internal switching mechanism that allows us to monitor and react to different cues *as if* simultaneously. But still, only one item at any one moment can be attended to. Processing occurs so quickly in real-life activities that momentary lags in the operation of the human system may be difficult to detect.

If it's true that only one item can be attended to and effectively responded to at one time, then attention to the right cue at the right time is extremely important, especially in externally-paced tasks. Owing to our limited information-processing capacities, attention must be restricted if those timely, quick, and accurate movements required in many sports are to be made.

But doesn't it appear that in reality we can do more than one thing at a time? Have you ever driven a car a distance on an uncrowded highway while thinking about personal problems and before you know it, you've covered ten miles? You might not even remember driving the car or any scenery or signs passed. It's as if the car were driven *automatically!*

In the *multi-channel model*, an alternative hypothesis to the single-channel model, it is proposed that we have the capability to attend to a few things simultaneously, under certain conditions. Generally speaking, consideration is given to:

(1) the nature of the cues to be responded to as well as the nature of the responses.

(2) the level of skill attained in performing one or more of the acts.

(3) the effort generated toward attending to one or both tasks.

On the first point, different information that does not come in via the same input channel places less attentional demand on the person. Relatively simple responses that use different output channels also require less attention. It is possible to perform two tasks together under such conditions, with no difference in achievement as compared to when such tasks are performed separately.

On the second point, a well-learned act is said to be *automatized* when it can be executed attention-free. Conscious attention is unnecessary. Since our limited channel capacity is not being tapped, a second act, one that might require conscious attention, can be performed at the same time. Our example earlier of driving a car while attending to thoughts of other mattters is a good example. The highly skilled basketball player, who dribbles a basketball while visually scanning the court and developing a passing or shooting strategy is another example.

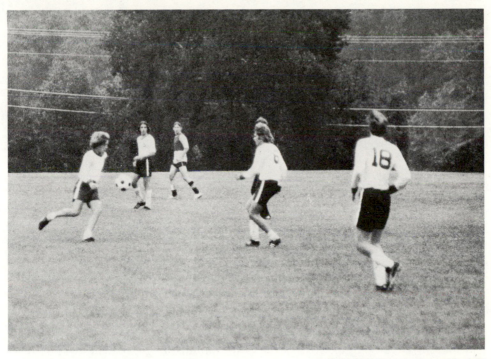

Featherkill Studios, Burnsville, MN

Attentional focus will change within a sport, depending on what's happening at the moment.

In the third case, effort is perceived as taking up attentional space. In other words, regardless of the apparent difficulty of a task or two of them, how much effort is allocated to either or one will be a determinant of one's ability to perform both of them effectively.

The nature of some tasks is to demand attention, to mobilize effort. Others may need effort, even though they don't actually demand it. Some difficult tasks seem to require neither. Two difficult tasks cannot be performed together if both are demanding and require personal effort. Most likely, as skill is acquired, tasks demand less effort on our part.

Practical Considerations

The teacher can make an activity analysis of the most relevant cues that need to be attended to at various stages of learning the activity. An analysis of the learners will indicate their skill level. When the student's level of skill is considered along with the nature of the activity, the teacher can isolate and emphasize the most important cues at any moment. Once the learner has succeeded in a particular situation, the teacher can administer the next level of cues. This process can continue as the learner achieves more and more.

Most teachers have a tendency to over-teach—to present too much information and too many cues at one time—either before or during a student's performance. This procedure can confuse and frustrate the learner. Information-processing capabilities are more limited in children and beginning mature learners, as compared to highly-skilled mature people. There is just so much information that a student can deal with any given time:

(1) too many cues will *overload* the system
(2) too little information will *underload* the system, leading to inattentiveness and loss of motivation

What does this mean in terms of instructional strategies? An adult who is presented with an irrelevant cue while trying to learn a task will pay only brief attention to it. Not so a young child: the child has not yet learned how to differentiate among cues. An irrelevant stimulus lengthens the time it takes the child to make a decision. The teacher, then, must realize this limitation, and the instructional strategy must reflect this realization. How? The teacher must present a learning environment free of irrelevant cues or else prompt the learner when necessary. Of course, with experience and maturity, the child will learn to control his or her perceptual and cognitive mechanisms. But the child must be guided toward this perception.

AROUSAL

Arousal is related to attention and is also associated with emotions. Arousal is the state of activation in an organism. In principle, there is an optimum level of arousal for each person in every activity. The ideal level of arousal varies with the situation and from person to person.

An under-aroused student may not pay attention to appropriate cues, and in general will not be highly motivated. An over-aroused student may also attend to the wrong cues; "trying too hard" naturally results in a breakdown of effective responses. How does the teacher determine the appropriate arousal level? This level for any circumstance depends on what is being demanded of the learner. Extremely complex activities require a relatively low level of arousal, because sensitive stimulus detection is necessary to respond to a complex array of stimuli, and a person in a highly aroused state cannot emit complex responses effectively. Simpler tasks, in which the movement is somewhat mechanical and for which speed or power (throwing a shot, for example) is primary, require higher levels of arousal.

Anxiety is one cause of arousal, and different people come to the same situation with different emotional levels. Obviously, then, a sensitive balance of ideal arousal for a particular activity must be worked out for each individual. To do this, the teacher must make a thorough task analysis to determine the nature of the situational demands and the response requirements on the part of each learner.

AROUSAL AND PERFORMANCE

Back in 1908, the Yerkes-Dodson "law" was formulated in which it was suggested that there is an optimal level of personal arousal or motivation to achieve in each activity. Many years later the *inverted-U hypothesis* was generated, which basically perpetuated same idea, but in a much more formal context.

Putting it simply, too little or too much arousal will be detrimental to achievement; just the right amount is desirable. The illustration of this point would look like this:

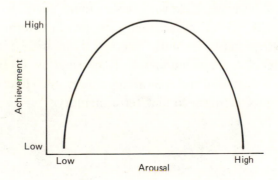

The optimal level of arousal necessary for each task will vary. Generally speaking, too little arousal reflects low motivation and possible inattention to appropriate cues, as well as slow and inappropriate movement decisions. Excessive arousal could cause non-flexibility and poor adaption in attention, as well as a breakdown in coordinated responses. The optimal level suggests the readiness to handle the demands of the activity accurately and efficiently.

Simple, repetitive, and power activities require more arousal and effort. Complex, intricate, and refined movement activities demand less arousal and effort. Thus, the nature of the activity suggests the appropriate arousal level.

SHORT- AND LONG-TERM MEMORY

It is popular in the field of psychology to talk in terms of two memory systems: Short-term and long-term. The *short-term* storage system receives information from the perceptual mechanism and then organizes it for decision-making purposes or for future storage. When information enters this system, it is rehearsed and processed temporarily. Short-term memory has been called the working memory. It is possible to transform information so as to free the individual to work on additional information. The better an individual can organize and process information here, the more functional he or she can be in complex activities. The activity in short-term memory, which includes the processing of incoming information along with reference to that which has been stored in long-term memory, determines a specific program of action.

Information that is properly organized and processed over a period of time can be transmitted from short-term memory to *long-term* memory. It remains there, in storage, to be retrieved at a later date as a comparison base to use for an analysis of present task demands (a reference point). Stored in long-term memory are knowledges, representations of skill, and meaningful experiences in general. We can think of them as being neatly compartmentalized there, waiting to be retrieved with the right cue. The more organized the information storage and the more efficient the retrieval process, the more likely it is that present actions will be compatible with achievement goals.

Remember that not all information goes into long-term memory. People respond quickly to present demands, meeting them with a sense of urgency and with no concern for maintaining that information in the system. Only when information is rehearsed and organized properly, for a long enough duration, will it proceed from short-term to long-term memory.

MOVEMENT PROGRAMS

The action in short-term memory generates a movement program. It is a plan of action, or a *schema*. The schema sends commands to the appropriate musculature, to prepare it for the forthcoming movement.

The more developed the movement program, the more effective the motor behavior will be. Less-skilled individuals have lower-order programs; with greater skill and experience, higher-order programs can be developed. These programs contain many subroutines of actions that appear to be executed almost subcon-

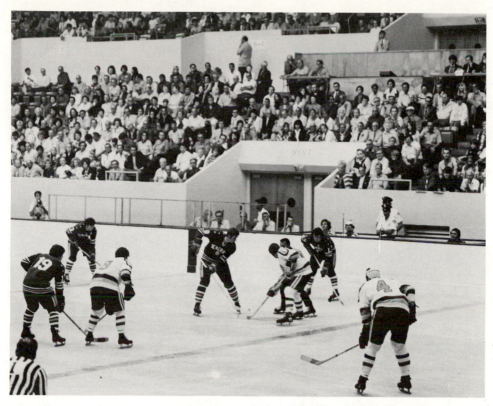

City News Bureau, St. Petersburg, Florida

In many sport situations, decisions leading to "movement programs" must be made very quickly.

sciously. These automatic activities free the conscious system to attend to other cues; they also help the learner to anticipate other cues.

The movement program identifies the specific characteristics of the intended response: location, distance, energy to be expended, amplitude, and speed; for example, the clearer its definition of these characteristics, the more likely it is that the movement will be compatible with situational demands.

You may find it hard to believe that so much information can be decided on in the human system in such a short period of time, and that somehow the person can control the response. The human system is unbelievably complex. Still, the full potential for achievement is very rarely, if ever, realized by performers. The challenge is obvious, then. There are ways to improve the students' processing capabilities as well as their decision-making processes. If the teacher uses the right technique, student performance can become even more skilled.

FEEDBACK

Once a movement is performed, various sense organs are activated that provide potential information to the student. *Response-produced feedback* is the information that is available to the learner as a result of his or her performance. Seeing and feeling help to provide information that can regulate ongoing acts or facilitate the performance in subsequent, related acts.

In most activities, a sufficient amount of response-produced information is available for the learner to evaluate and to apply to the learning situation. Good learners use feedback to their advantage. However, there are certain activities in which personal feedback is limited. In gymnastics and diving, for example, it is difficult for the student to know how a movement looked. Here, external sources of information—a coach, a videotape—are necessary.

The ultimate goal is to make learners as self-dependent as possible. Most beginners are externally dependent; they rely on the instructor's guidance and depend too much on information in the environment. With experience and improved skill they become more self-reliant. That is, they learn how to use the most appropriate feedback information in an effective way, helping to improve their performances on the basis of this information. The teacher can help the learners to become better self-managers, encouraging them to assess their own performance instead of relying on external guidance.

Figure 7–1 illustrated the basic processes that are described in this section. From the time information—either external or internal in source—is recognized, a series of complex operations occurs that leads to the intended movement goal. More complicated acts require more sophisticated processing of information. The model of motor behavior presented here is a general one. The flow of information is similar for all people (barring a handicap), although the quality of the processing will differ, depending on the strategies that each individual uses in order to control and transmit information. There are other factors that can also lead to differences in learning and performance.

FACTORS THAT INFLUENCE LEARNER PROCESSES

Growth and Development

As children develop, their maturational readiness to acquire more complex skills grows as well. Differences in age and experience do create different capabilities. Young or inexperienced learners are somewhat restricted in the ways in

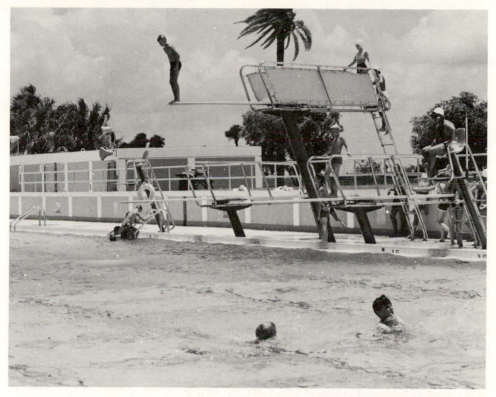

City News Bureau, St. Petersburg, Florida

With growth and development, learner capabilities improve.

which they can acquire skills: They must learn techniques to process information as well as have the means to control the coordination of their musculature. The phenomenon occurs with older people as well. As people age, limitations in their information-processing capabilities can impede performance in more complex tasks. Thus developmental factors certainly play a role in the ability of the human system to acquire and perform skills.

Structural and Functional Capabilities

The ability to perform well depends, too, on the person's physical structure. If the sense organs, the musculature, or any part of the nervous system are not in good operating order, it is difficult to perform more complex motor skills adequately. Although various compensatory mechanisms can operate, in many situations they are not sufficient to help learners achieve proficiency.

Other physical elements—strength and endurance, for example—should be present as required by the demands of a given activity. The variation among students in regard to their physical states of conditioning is another factor in differing performances.

Cognitive and Psychological Factors

Intellectual ability within the normal range of intelligence does not relate too much to motor-skill performance. Research does indicate that mentally handicapped children have more difficulty in learning complex motor skills. They need special instructional consideration, and even then they will probably be slightly behind in their achievement of motor skills.

However, psychological factors—motivations, attitudes, and expectations—play a large part in learning. One of the biggest disappointments for many teachers is the realization that not all the students who enter a classroom or a gymnasium are highly motivated to learn. The effective teacher must think of ways to energize these students, to put them in the right frame of mind for learning. Students have to want to learn if they are going to learn to any meaningful degree.

Situational Conditions

The ability to learn and perform skills will vary, depending on the conditions in which the learning takes place. A proper environment is conducive to motivation and learning. Some conditions are more advantageous than others. Lighting, acoustics, and temperature, for example, play a part in performance.

There are, of course, situational factors that the teacher cannot control: elevation (mountain versus sea level), climate, and weather conditions, for example. But certain conditions can be more favorable than others for the learning of certain activities, and they should be considered in the instructional program. These conditions include space—an optimal class size for the space available—and adequate equipment.

Social and Cultural Influences

Attitudes toward specific activities vary from society to society. Soccer is very popular in Europe; football in the United States; ice hockey in Canada; and swimming in Australia. The popularity of certain sports in a particular

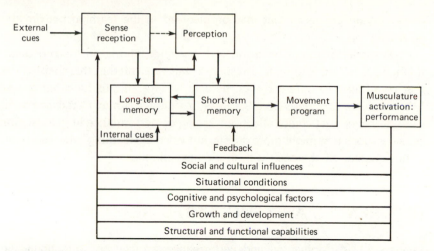

FIGURE 7–2. Individuals differ in performance potential and learning capabilities due to a variety of factors, as exemplified here. (From R. N. Singer and W. Dick, *Teaching physical education: A systems approach,* 2d ed. Boston: Houghton Mifflin, 1980.)

society may very well influence the attitudes and choices of young people in that society.

The impact of culture is not to be taken lightly. Not only does it influence activity preference; it also acts on activity persistence. In some cultures, achievement in sport is admired, and participants, knowing this, work harder. In other countries, sport has a lower priority, and as a result, fewer young people train intensively. Even in the same country, we can see regional attitudes toward and preferences for different physical activities.

Figure 7–2 shows the impact of these additional considerations on the potential for students to learn and to perform motor skills.

SUMMARY

As viewed from an information processing perspective, a series of operations or processes becomes activated within a person from signal selection to response execution. How effectively these processes function will influence the quality of learning and performance.

Human capabilities and capacities have theoretical limits, but appropriate strategies can enhance the operations that occur within such limitations. The quality and appropriateness of a motor response or a series of them depends upon the way sensory, perceptual, memorial, decision-making, and feedback processes operate. Attention and arousal have the potential to influence any one or many processes that may be involved in the learning/performance of an activity.

A model of motor behavior, with heavy emphasis on the processes that might be activated leading to a response, was presented in this chapter. Factors that could lead to differences in the way we are able to function, or wish to function, were also described. Whereas in Chapter 6 many practice conditions were proposed that could influence learning or performance in general, practice considerations that might more directly influence the learning processes indicated in this chapter will be dealt with in the next chapter.

REFERENCES AND SUGGESTED READINGS

Landers, D. M. Motivation and performance: arousal and attentional factors. In W. F. Straub (ed.), *Sport psychology: an analysis of athlete behavior,* second edition. Ithaca, N.Y.: Mouvement Publications, 1980.

Marteniuk, R. *Information processing in motor skills.* New York: Holt, Rinehart and Winston, 1976.

Singer, R. N. *Motor learning and human performance,* third edition. New York: Macmillan Publishing Co., Inc., 1980, Chapter 6.

Singer, R. N. Motor skills and learning strategies. In O'Neill, W. F. (ed.), *Learning strategies.* New York: Academic Press, 1978.

Underwood, G. Attentional selectivity and behavioral control. In Underwood, G. (ed.), *Strategies of information processing.* New York: Academic Press, 1978.

INFLUENCING
THE LEARNER

Meaningful practice produces effective learning outcomes. We as teachers or coaches can impact upon learners in various positive ways. We can help them to improve the way those learners' processes involved in learning operate. We can establish conditions favorable to learning, those that bear on motivation.

Most, if not all, learning in formal programs should be potentially useful in the future. It would be desirable if such learning were retained at a reasonable level for a reasonable period of time. Similarly, it would be nice if we could apply present learnings to future related situations. In the first case, we were talking about retention, and in the second case, transfer. Both are important potential outcomes of learning; both can be influenced by the way initial practice conditions are established and learning processes are activated and applied.

We will examine in this chapter concepts, research, and practical ideas related to motivation, supplementary feedback (knowledge of results of performance), transfer, and retention. Through the use of effective instructional and learning techniques, the acquisition, retention, and transfer of motor skills should be enhanced. But personal motivation underlies any potential for success. So does feedback availability. Therefore, we will first take a look at how motivation works and how it can be influenced. After a discussion on supplementary feedback, we will analyze retention and transfer and ways to improve the likelihood of both.

MAKING PRACTICE MEANINGFUL

As a reminder from before, good practice leads to good learning. Our two obligations are to (1) understand the activities we wish to teach and how they might be taught best, and (2) understand the nature of the learning process, how students in general learn, and where there are important individual differences to consider.

Practice can be meaningful when it is organized and managed scientifically and logically to the satisfaction of a teacher. Practice must be meaningful as interpreted by the learners.

UNDERSTANDING MOTIVATION

Motivation is such a complex phenomenon that it's often difficult to understand how it affects decisions and behavior; on many occasions it may not be clear why we do or want to do certain things. Yet being motivated often implies wanting to achieve certain goals, goals that may gratifying our needs. Motivation influences what we do (if there is a choice), how long we do it, and how well we do it.

Selection of an Activity

There are more hours available to us than we realize to use as we wish. Preferences are developed. Activities that are personally gratifying or will be rewarded in some way are usually decided upon. Whatever the reason, in a free-choice situation, the activities that we decide to participate in reflect motivations toward those activities. Obviously, the more a person is motivated to learn a particular activity, the more he or she will practice at it, even if given alternative possibilities.

Persistence at Practice

As was just stated, practice is sustained, if it is optional to practice, when motivation to do so is present. Improvement in complex motor activities is associated with extensive and intensive training, proficiency does not come easily. The extent of practice will necessarily depend upon the individual's achievement goals and personal capabilities for the particular activity.

Optimization for Performance

Motivation levels immediately prior to and during performance need to be optimal. The same was said about attention and arousal. Thought and emotional processes should be "tuned" appropriately for the demands of the activity, considering the personal characteristics of the individual.

Sometimes motivation (state of activation) needs to be relatively high, as in power events. Sometimes this state should be relatively low, as in precision and control events, like hitting a golf ball. Lifting a heavy weight, throwing a projectile as far as possible, and swimming or running an event as quickly as possible, are examples of acts that can be mechanized and that require maximal effort yield. A highly aroused (but controlled) state is desirable. Shooting at a target, executing a foul shot, or rolling a bowling ball are activities that demand great influence over emotions, leading to refined movement control. The attainment of an optimal motivational state just before and during performance can be learned with practice. The old saying, "The more motivation the better," is obviously not true in many cases. What is true is that many times athletes are over-motivated and subsequently perform worse than they should; they need to be less aroused.

Remember, *higher* levels of motivation lead to greater probabilities of selection of, persistence at, and effort in an activity. Motivation appropriate *(optimal)* to the nature of the demands of the activity will lead to better performance in that activity.

INTRINSIC AND EXTRINSIC MOTIVATION

Many reasons may be offered as to why people do what they do. They have often been categorized as *intrinsic* (internal) or *extrinsic* (external) sources of motivation. Usually associated with internal motivation is doing something for fun, to develop skills, or to become fulfilled. Extrinsic motivation is typically associated with being engaged in an activity in order to gain materialistically, for rewards, or for recognition. The attempt to achieve in a particular sport, as in any endeavor, may involve both types of motivation, but they may be unequal as forces of influence in a person. Both kinds, independently or together, will determine behavior. Let us first analyze situations in which a sense of inner direction and commitment needs to be developed within an individual, which is the thrust of achievement motivation programs, and examine their effectiveness.

Afterwards, we will look at principles of shaping behavior with rewards and reinforcers, and the potential effectiveness of extrinsic sources of motivation on performance. As will be seen, it is possible for us to influence the dependency of others either toward external sources of motivation, *or* toward internal sources of motivation.

THE MOTIVATION TO ACHIEVE

In order to be internally motivated and stay that way certain personal conditions should be present. You have to give yourself direction. You have to feel and be in control—of yourself. You have to be optimistically realistic.

People who demonstrate a strong need to achieve tend to:

(1) set high, specific, and obtainable *goals*.
(2) arrange personal plans or *programs* that *will be followed* to help reach those goals.
(3) constantly *monitor* their *progress*, and if off course, modify or change goals, programs, or both.
(4) *think positively*.
(5) look to *personal factors* that might *cause* desired results, such as *effort*, rather than luck.
(6) *evaluate* what they have done *objectively*, and look to improve their effort rather than blame others or circumstances.

Of course, such a personal commitment plan can lead to materialistic rewards as well as self-satisfaction. Indeed, it often does. But to receive some degree of satisfaction from participation in an activity, a reasonable skill level usually helps. The improvement in skill is more likely to happen, and to happen expediently, if personal commitment is shown. To depend solely on rewards may result in short-sighted achievements. Yet, this is not to say that reward systems do not have their place. They can be very powerful influences on our behavior.

But let us consider here motivation that primarily comes from within one's self. Early in life, manifestations of intrinsic motivation are probably due to the need to be confident and self-determining in relation to one's environment. With development, the child's generalized intrinsic motivation is differentiated into specific motives. Still, it is commonly observed that most children enjoy physical challenges, a degree of risk-taking, and many forms of play.

UNDERACHIEVING

An underachiever is someone who achieves noticeably less than expected in some endeavor. A student who scores high on a mathematical aptitude test, does well during class discussions, and proceeds to fare poorly on a final examination, would be called an underachiever.

An athlete seems to possess many characteristics associated with achievement in a particular sport. During practice, progress is fine. Much is expected of him or her. Then, during the actual contest, performance is miserable. This athlete, too, is an underachiever.

Since people differ in many respects, such disappointments could be attributed to various factors detailed in the next chapter. One possibility is low motivation to achieve, and this topic will be discussed in the next chapter. Another likely one is poor test-taking ability for the student and poor contest competitive ability for the athlete. The stress of taking important tests, of being evaluated in important events, is more than some people can handle. Their feelings of anxiety become so great that their performance level does not come close to matching their true learning or skill level. As the famous motivational psychologist John Atkinson has stated, the true ability of the person who is less than optimally motivated will be underestimated by a test score. The true ability of the person who is more than optimally motivated, who is overmotivated given the requirements of the task, will similarly be underestimated.

With an understanding of how to identify feelings of high anxiety, and what to do about them, people could have more control over themselves. They would be better able to cope with situations. They could put themselves in more optimal states to demonstrate their accomplishments. Good achievers have learned how to ready themselves for tests, contests, and other types of performances. But in many cases, techniques might have to be taught. Many articles and books describing alternative approaches are available to assist people in reducing anxiety.

Due to cultural factors, educational programs, and reward systems, many children become interested in activities other than, or in addition to, play-type activities. If children are to sustain or even develop further an interest in motor skills, their intrinsic motivations for them should not be undermined. Motor activities need to be:

(1) Personally valued.
(2) Valued by others close to the child.
(3) Satisfying, challenging, and enjoyable.

When these factors, as well as the six qualities that high achievers seem to possess (listed earlier on page 156), are present, a person is most likely to have satisfying and successful experience in an activity. Martin Covington and Richard Beery (1976), in an excellent and insightful book, point out problems that children have in regard to motivation and achievement in school learning. The basic theme is that teachers should be more sensitive to the threatening learning environments that they themselves inadvertently create. These authors call for more situations that are frustration-free, that allow learners to attain feelings of success, attributed to personal effort. Teacher encouragement, rather than praise and criticism, which promote performance dependent on an external source, leads to personal feelings of self-direction and self-confidence.

As to the six considerations that lead to an achievement orientation, let's go into more depth about them. *Goal setting* has been discussed in another section. We need not discuss this type of motivational activity again except to re-emphasize the value of goal setting as a personal motivational tool to improve achievement.

Plans or *programs* to fulfill goals must be compatible with the goals. They should be realistic; they must be feasible. If there is commitment, the chances are the program will be successful in helping one to obtain the goals.

Next, *evaluation* must be an ongoing process. If everything is working, fine. If not, either the goals must be lowered or else the training program must be intensified. If there is an indication that one can surpass the established long-term goals, then a decision is an order: whether to retain the same goals anyway, or to raise the goals. At any rate, the continuous monitoring of progress is a necessity.

Throughout it all, a *positive outlook* should prevail. Positive attitudes, constructive self-evaluation, and a feeling that goals can be accomplished will increase the likelihood of their realization.

Consistent with this perspective is an *internalized feeling of control* over one's actions and outcomes. Julian Rotter pointed out a while ago that some of us are primarily internals and some are externals. Internals looks to themselves (ability and effort) to make things happen. Externals view the outside world (others and situations) as the major influences over their successes and failures. People who are more inner-directed have a better chance at succeeding.

Finally, once performance occurs, the evaluation of causative factors *(attributions)* to internal but unstable factors (like effort) is desirable. Attributional theory, popularized today mostly through the effort of Bernard Weiner (1974, 1980), has led to an abundance of research on the relationship of attributions (the reasons people give to themselves as to why they did what they did) to future

WHAT MOTIVATED YOU?

Think of an activity (preferably a sport) that you spent quite a lot of time practicing in order to become good. Now, reflect as to the major reason why you practiced and why you wanted to excel. Any other reasons? Did they change during the course of time, from the first time you practiced until the point when you stopped (if you stopped)? If you are still involved, consider the present.

Can you identify the source(s) of your motivation? Were they intrinsic or extrinsic? Both? Did it (they) change over time?

Think of two different activities in which you became involved, one primarily for intrinsic reasons and one primarily for extrinsic reasons. Were there differences in the satisfaction you received? How about continued level of interest? Did you practice longer each day and over time in the activity that was intrinsic versus the one that was extrinsic? Most educators and psychologists believe that internal sources of motivation lead to more satisfying experiences and accomplishments, that perseverance will be increased. Was this true in your situation?

Rewards can be helpful or harmful in situations regarding interest in and persistence at practice. In the latter case, research indicates that there may be an *undermining effect,* that is to say, many children may be internally interested in an activity at the start. They may find it challenging, stimulating, and enjoyable. Then, after a certain amount of experience, they are offered rewards for choosing and/or persisting at that same activity. The rewards have the potential of undermining intrinsic motivation, resulting in a lessened interest in and persistence at the activity!

Take youth sport programs, for instance. Many kids love to play in sport for the sake of playing. Then they join a program, let's say swimming, where prizes, ribbons, or trophies are given to winners of events in competition. Or they may be given to every participant, in graduated form, depending on their finish. Soon kids learn to depend on these rewards. They may swim for the rewards, rather than the fun or challenge of developing skills in swimming. If that happens, a promising swimming future may soon be terminated. Has something like this ever happened to you?

goal-level expectations when performance occurs again. In turn, they are related to achievement.

When all these factors operate, the chances of achieving have increased. Analyze yourself in learning situations. Do they operate for you?

ATTRIBUTIONS

Returning to the topic of attributions, it would be beneficial to explore this area a little further. Four major reasons people offer for their performances are (1) ability, (2) effort, (3) luck, or (4) the difficulty of the activity. The first two reasons are personal, or internal. The other two are situational, or external to the person.

Ability is a stable factor, and therefore is not controllable by the person during performance. If an individual perceives a stable factor as the cause for failure, he or she will probably fail again. An attribution of failure to effort (or rather the lack of it—during performance or practice leading to an event), is good because effort is unstable but controllable. As Weiner (1980) emphasizes, the major attribution that impairs the striving for achievement is a perception of low ability. An attribution to a lack of energy expenditure (effort) is the most adaptive attribution for failure. Instructors should help learners to ascribe poor performance to lack of effort rather than to luck or ability. They need to learn that they can influence their own outcomes; they can work harder to achieve more. Greater effort and practice leads to improved ability, and consequently better results.

THE ENVIRONMENT

The instructor controls the learning environment and the learning procedures. Merely constantly changing a learning or working situation from day to day may enhance learning or productivity, or at least help to maintain acceptable levels of output. The same type of practice under the same conditions day after day can be boring and monotonous, but changing drills or learning experiences, and modifying learning environments, can be stimulating and motivating.

This was shown to be true many years ago in the famous Hawthorne studies. Workers were studied for a long period of time in an industrial plant. Many factors were observed. One of the major conclusions was that by simply modifying the working environment of the people (such as painting the walls, changing light fixtures), production was maintained or increased over time. The people were more excited about coming to work. They looked forward to seeing what was new. They felt that somebody was taking an interest in them. Ironically, none of the environmental modifications should have had any bearing on productivity. But psychologically, they had their impact on the workers.

REWARDS AS MOTIVATORS

Rewards systems, events that occur from sources external to a person, can be effective in causing those people with a low interest to participate in an activity or to excel in it. They can help to attract individuals to activities or to encourage their practice in them.

Rewards or punishments given after an act inform the person what should be done or shouldn't be done in a particular situation. They can shape behaviors when administered appropriately. We will discuss the nature of reinforcers and reinforcement theory shortly. For now, however, we can see that (1) Rewards can be *incentives* to participate, practice, and achieve; and (2) Rewards can *shape behaviors* toward a certain direction.

Indeed, much research evidence as well as everyday experiences and observations support these conclusions. Two major considerations with regard to rewards are (1) The degree to which they are *interpreted* as such by those to whom

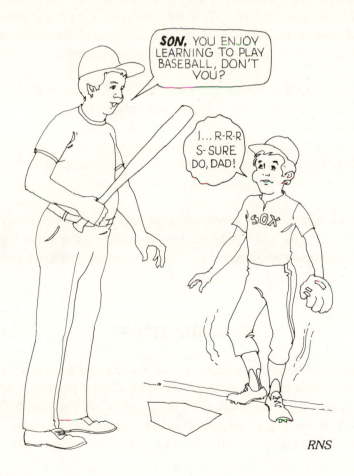

RNS

they are administered; and (2) The degree to which they are *relied on* for interest in and perseverance at an activity.

In the first situation, the same object may not possess the same incentive properties for different people. A five-dollar bill means a lot to a child in poverty but may be of little perceived value to a "rich kid." Therefore, if rewards are to be used in learning situations, they should be analyzed carefully for their potential value to the learners. Rewards are used often in sport in recognition for good performances. If children come to expect selective rewards (stars on football helmets, names posted on locker room boards), then these criteria should be understood by all so as not to disappoint those who do not receive rewards but feel they deserve recognition for their efforts. And, of course, mere verbal encouragement by a coach to an athlete or a teacher to a student for a job well done can be a very effective motivational technique.

In the second case, complete dependence on external rewards for what we do is not considered to be desirable. External sources of motivation, it is true, can augment internal sources. Both can and probably do operate to some relative degree in most athletes. Many cultures place a high premium on externally-applied rewards to shape the behaviors of its members. More ideal would be the establishment of settings and programs that encourage:

(1) Inner direction toward participation in physical activities;
(2) The realization of the value of these experiences;
(3) The continual quest for self-improvement, self-competence, self-fulfillment, self-realization; and
(4) Challenges that can contribute to the realization of potential means of expression, skill, knowledge, and enjoyment.

Cognitive and affective behaviors must be tapped more often. External reinforcers, commands, and "blind" following would appear to be less desirable in the long run for these purposes.

REINFORCEMENT

Through the scientific and systematic use of rewards and punishments administered in various ways to rats learning mazes and other tasks, many implications have been drawn as to the shaping of behaviors of all organisms. Behaviorist B. F. Skinner is given greatest credit for the advancement of the theory of instrumental conditioning. On the basis of the activity demonstrated by an

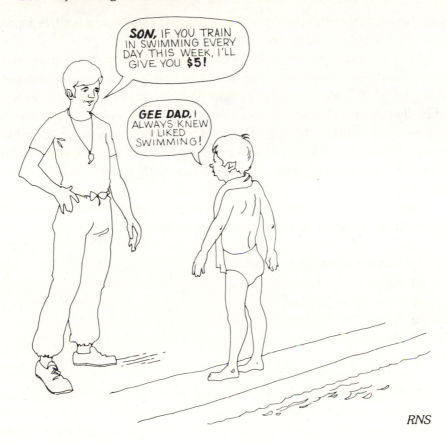

RNS

organism, he suggested that reinforcers would inform the organism as to the appropriateness of its behavior.

A *reinforcer* is anything that increases the probability of the occurrence of a certain act or behavior. *Positive reinforcers* follow upon the demonstration of desirable behaviors and are themselves desirable to the subject; hence they are instrumental in shaping behaviors. Naturally, this is the intention behind the use of awards. If the *disappearance* of a stimulus as a consequence of a response results in an increased possibility that the response *will* occur again, the withdrawn stimulus is called a *negative reinforcer*.

Punishment is an *aversive stimulus* that may follow a response in order to reduce or eliminate it. Punishment, let us remember, tells us what *not* to do, not what to do. The lack of reinforcers or the administration of some form of punishment can help to distinguish behavioral tendencies; the provision of reinforcers can help to promote the repetition of ideal behaviors or to shape behaviors in an ideal direction. Although punishments can be effective, they can also be a source of frustration and bitterness. They represent a negative approach in dealing with others. Positive reinforcers constitute a positive approach and are prefereable in most, but not all, situations.

Many behavior modification programs are based on these principles of reinforcement. Such programs have been used advantageously to help people curb antisocial, delinquent, and other undesirable behaviors. Individuals can also modify their own behaviors if they possess sufficient will and direction. But many find this process difficult. Thus, external applicators serve to influence personal attitudes and thought patterns. Once they are of sufficient magnitude and conviction, personal resources can operate without the need for external reinforcers.

With regard to the utilization of reinforcers, researchers have consideration given to the schedule of administering these as to:

(1) frequency (variable or fixed),
(2) ratio,
(3) interval,
(4) type,
(5) magnitude.

As to the *frequency* with which reinforcers may be applied, too much or too little will probably both be relatively ineffective. The optional amount needs to be determined. But the belief that more reinforcement is better is probably overstated, especially if the reinforcement is administered in a constantly predictable manner. Consider a baseball batter. If he got a hit every time at bat the activity would probably become boring; there would be no challenge. And no hits would lead to frustration and disappointment. But to obtain three hits out of every ten at bat, and not know when they will occur or what kinds of hits they will be, leads to feelings of being satisfied and challenged.

Speaking of not knowing for sure when a reinforcer will be applied (in batting, let's say, when a hit will occur), it appears that a predetermined reinforcement *ratio*—ratio of reinforcers to nonreinforcers after an act—is not as effective as a non-predetermined ratio. With regard to *intervals*, the more immediately the reinforcer follows the act, the better. In this way no additional activity can occur before receipt of the reinforcer. It is of greatest impact when administered right after the person performs the act.

Reinforcers can be of many *types*. Sometimes they can be redundant or complementary in the same situation, such as a baseball player getting a hit, receiving praise from the coach and other players, and reading about it in the newspapers. If only one type of reinforcement is used, the one thought to be most effective with each person should be determined. In some cases, it is felt that most people will respond similarly to a particular reinforcer; in other cases potential reinforcers may be valued differently by individuals.

Similarly, most people will respond more favorably to reinforcers of a greater *magnitude*. At least they will initially. Of course, sometimes magnitude is of absolute value, in that most everyone would interpret it the same way; at other times magnitude is of relative value, in that personal perspectives make for individualized interpretations. Salaries for professional baseball players assume absolute values; the quantity of praise received may be responded to differentially.

The things we do or say to others after they have performed in an activity may be reinforcing. They may be motivating. They may be informational. In other words, they may provide feedback about performance to the learner in addition to that which is present for him or her from personal efforts and available sources.

SUPPLEMENTING FEEDBACK

Earlier in this material, in talking about the human behaving system, reference was made to feedback, its importance and role in learning. Often information is present to the learner through her or his senses during or after performance, or both, as to the adequacy of that performance; that information is feedback. Certainly in the early stages of learning it's a necessity. Learning cannot occur without it.

But on many occasions that feedback is inadequate for the purposes of the learner. Or it may be adequate but the learner does not use it effectively. Under such circumstance, *supplementary*, or *augmented*, *feedback* will be necessary. This type of feedback is feedback provided from an external source—an object or a person—to the learner. Remember, if the student has a sufficient amount of information available from his or her own efforts, and knows how to use it, supplementary feedback is redundant and unnecessary. But it may serve to reinforce or motivate. The important consideration is to analyze activities and learners, and the possible need for supplementary feedback. Then you might try to determine when such feedback is potentially informational, reinforcing, or motivational (and what purpose this feedback might serve).

Knowledge of Results

The expression *knowledge of results* has been used synonymously with the term *feedback*. In this material and for clarification purposes, it is recommended that the term *feedback* be associated with self-generated information about one's

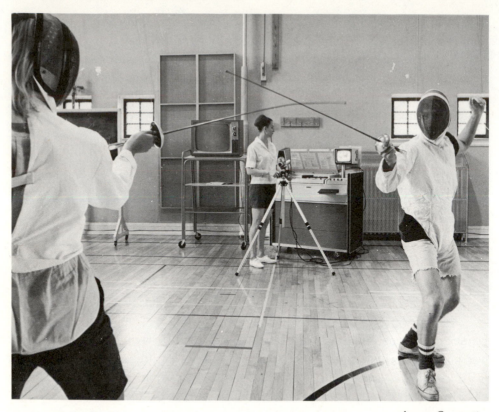

Ampex Corporation

Students being videotaped as they fence, with the information to be used as supplementary feedback as soon as they are finished.

performance and the results of it. *Supplementary feedback* will be interpreted similarly as knowledge of results *(KR)*. An abundance of literature is readily available on the role of KR in learning various types of tasks. In more recent years, distinctions have been made in the motor learning literature between the terms *knowledge of results (KR)* of a performance and *knowledge about the performance (KP)* itself. *KR* refers to information presented to the learner about the outcome of his/her performances, for example, an arrow in the target.

Knowledge About Performance

Information can and should be provided to the person about the nature of his/her performance. Outcome is one thing; the means to the outcome another matter. Techniques, strategies, skills, form, and other considerations during a

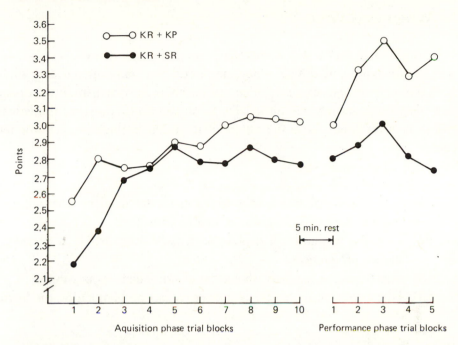

Figure 8–1. Performance comparisons between two groups that received knowledge of results *(KR),* one with knowledge of performance *(KP)* in addition, the other with social reinforcement *(SR).* (From S. A. Wallace, and R. W. Hagler, Knowledge of performance and the learning of a closed motor skill. *Research Quarterly,* 1979, 50, 265–271.)

movement action or a lengthy activity can be analyzed, and this information can then be provided to the learner. Again, consideration must be given to the intrinsic availability of such information, and any need for KP.

Wallace and Hagler (1979) designed a study in which the importance of *KP* was examined. Two groups of subjects had to learn to shoot a basketball with their non-dominant hands ten feet from the basket. Both groups were given *KR* during the acquisition blocks of trials. One group, in addition, received *KP* (information about execution). The other group was administered social reinforcement *(SR)* in the form of verbal encouragement. In the next phase of the study, for five blocks of trials only *KR* was given to these groups. *KP* and *SR* were withheld. As can be seen in Figure 8–1, the group that had earlier received *KP* was more successful than the *SR* group. As pointed out by Wallace and Hagler "There are many skills, such as throwing a projectile with accuracy, where learning the proper mechanics of the movement early in skill acquisition may be as important as producing the desired outcome" (p. 271).

When and Why

Considering *KP* and *KR* together, we may raise many questions as to their nature, type, and timing. They may *offered* or *administered concurrently* (during an activity) or *terminally*. The *medium* may be visual, auditory, or some other means. If administered terminally, feedback can be provided immediately or at some later time. As to the *nature* of it, it can be highly precise or more general.

Such alternatives suggest:

(1) A task analysis, and a determination of the need or possibilities for ongoing feedback or terminal feedback, or both.
(2) That the medium will depend on what's available, convenience, and learner preferences.
(3) That terminal feedback should be as immediate as possible.
(4) That feedback should be as specific as can be handled by the learner.

PROMOTING TRANSFER

One of the greatest hindrances to learning a so-called "new" activity is the lack of perception on the learner's part of the relationship of the now with the then. Many past learnings and experiences can be tied in to present intended learnings. It is rare, if ever, that we learn a totally new skill after our early formative years.

The study of the effect of past learnings on present ones, or present ones on previous ones, is called *transfer*, or the *transfer of learning*. In a laboratory setting, we can take two related tasks and determine the degree of influence one task has on the learning of the other. In fact, the degree of relationship can be established between input type and availability, information processing demands, and response choices.

When one type of experience (such as learning a particular task) promotes the learning of a task, it is considered to be an indication of *positive transfer*. If it hinders learning, it is called *negative transfer;* if there is absolutely no influence, it is referred to as *zero transfer*. In the laboratory, we can analyze the relationship of one activity to another, and the possible transfer effects of what has been learned in one activity to that which needs to be learned in another activity.

But real-world activities are not as easy to speculate accurately about. For instance, sports activities are very complex and involve the learning of many skills and strategies, and it's not as easy to suggest the effect of learning from one sports skill or strategy to another as it might be with laboratory tests. Laboratory tests are usually much simpler and easier to control in their administration. Does the learning of tennis facilitate the learning of badminton? Racketball? How about basketball? Do skills acquired in it aid in the acquisition of volleyball skills? Does a good baseball swing promote the development of a good golf stroke?

These are sample questions. Many more could be raised. But how would you answer the example questions just raised? Let's take the tennis/badminton example. On the positive side, both sports involve tracking a projectile and contacting it with a racket. Strategies in both sports as to moving the opponent are somewhat similar. Even many of the strokes appear to be fairly similar, although on a technical level, they are not. On the negative side, badminton is a wrist sport: stroking in many situations require good wrist action. In tennis stroking very often should not involve wrist action: the racket is an extension of the arm, and the ball should be hit with the wrist firm. Footwork is not so important in badminton; it is in tennis. The projectiles, rackets, court dimensions, and movements are somewhat dissimilar in the two sports.

In the beginning, transfer effects are general. But specific practice in techniques and skills, as well as the development of the appropriate conditioning level, will determine higher levels of skill, be the person a former tennis player or not. If the non-tennis player is in the same physical condition as the tennis player, he or she may eventually out-perform the tennis player, as the tennis player will have to first unlearn certain performance behaviors before the correct behavior will set in. Every sport requires specific patterns of movement in specific situations, and the refinement of skill requires highly specialized training. Remember too that, as skill improves, practice should *simulate* ultimate potential test (contest) conditions whenever possible. More experience under "real" settings prepares the student for possible situations and how to respond in them. Transfer effects are most positive when practice conditions and test conditions are similar. When going to take a classroom test, prepare by taking it home under test-like conditions (guessing what kinds of questions will be asked, and writing them out within the specified time allotment). Many people overestimate what they know. In the classroom environment, knowing not only means knowing, but showing. A performance test will reflect what the student presumably knows. Therefore, following test procedures within time constraints is as important as knowledge of the class material.

The same is true in sports. Practice in artificial, controlled settings may not prepare the athlete adequately for an event. Practice under pressure while getting tired may come closer. Each sport has its own considerations for practice in this regard.

So, what might we expect? It appears that the learning of tennis can help as well as hinder the learning of badminton, all skills and strategies considered. Since it has been shown in laboratory tests that positive transfer is more powerful than negative transfer, I am going to assume that people who can play tennis at a reasonably level of proficiency will fare better *at first* when attempting to acquire badminton skills than people who have never played tennis or who play tennis rather poorly.

To conduct an experiment on this problem, we would form two groups of non-badminton players, one half of whom could pass a tennis skill test indicating reasonable experience and competency. The other half would consist of non-tennis players. Then both groups of subjects would be taught, in exactly the same manner, to play badminton. The groups of subjects might be compared in achievement in (1) badminton skills tests, (2) form while playing in a game, and (3) rankings in a class tournament after all had competed against each other. If tennis experience did make a difference, then the two groups should be about even in these measures. If one group were better or worse than the other, then this difference would be attributed to prior tennis-playing experience.

What Influences What

As can be seen, previous learnings can influence present learnings, depending on their relationship(s). But what specifically needs to be considered? In older or more traditional psychology, the nature of the stimulus/i and response(s) would be analyzed in a previously learned task and a to-be-learned task. If stimuli and responses were somewhat similar, positive transfer should result. If stimuli are different but responses are the same, we would still expect positive transfer. If the stimuli were the same but the response is different, negative transfer should have occurred. If both stimuli and responses are dissimilar, then zero transfer would be expected.

As mentioned before, laboratory tests can be simplified and controlled so that stimulus-response possibilities and relationships between tasks are easily identified. However, in real-life activities like sports many factors operate. Relationships between activities are not so easily clarified. And, as realized more and more, although acts are somewhat specifically refined for specific situations, *learning strategies* may be more generalizable across tasks. *Processes* that need to be used to achieve in different categories of tasks may be similar.

Capabilities related to problem solving, anticipation, concentration, relaxation, motivation, and readiness to learn/perform, for example, can be useful in many situations. They have to be (1) learned well in terms of the "skills" involved; and (2) applied correctly in subsequent task learning/performance contexts. In the second case, recognition of situations that need the activation of well-learned self-directed processes will enhance the use of such capabilities. Therefore, the first step is to identify the nature of the learning situation and personal resources needed. Then they must be applied.

Thus, it is apparent that transfer can involve the present with the past as to (1) the recognition of task characteristics and demands, (2) the use of personal resources appropriate to accomplish the task, and (3) the activation of movement actions.

Another type of question may be asked. To what degree will performance in one activity influence performance in another related one, when both are well-learned? Let's say you just played racketball and have enough energy to play tennis. Would your tennis game be messed up? Most likely, only at first, and for a little while. Timing will be off briefly as one gets used to the new situational context and the demands of the activity. *Interference* with skill transfer is least likely between two tasks when the acts or activities are well-learned.

Generality versus Specificity Issues

Throughout the century, the pendulum has swung back and forth as to conceptual and practical beliefs about the nature of transfer. When Thorndike formulated his Identical Elements Theory in the early 1900s, curricula in the schools were changed drastically. For instance, courses in logic were dropped, as there were no evidence that logic learned in the classroom could be applied to daily situations in which logic and common sense might be involved. Course content and experiences were considered to be somewhat specialized and non-generalizable.

But in the 1920s to the 1940s, as we examine major publications in education, psychology, and physical education, many tests were developed to assess general intelligence, personality traits, and general motor ability. It was felt that generalized tests could predict behaviors and achievements in specific areas. Such tests were moderately successful. Other efforts suggested generalized transfer possibilities from some learnings to others. But still other efforts tended to remind us of the unique processes we possess in regard to achievement in each activity, such as the fact that the rate of learning for each person is a function of the task itself rather than a generalizable capability across all kinds of tasks.

Things really became confusing for physical educators in the 1960s. On one hand, influential Franklin Henry and his students were apparently demonstrating the independence of performances in various motor tasks, and advocated a Theory of Neuromotor Specificity. Yet, believers in movement education and problem-solving techniques were saying that "understandings" are transferable in reasonably related contexts. So where are we today?

Probably, somewhere in the middle. In other words, we obviously do not learn each act in isolation. Acts are learned in contexts. Learning processes, strategies, and skills can be applied to related acts and situations. Each learning experience is not and need not be considered as truly new.

And yet, we should not overestimate the potential of past learnings to be generalizable in present learning situations. Every skill, within and between sports, for example, requires very distinct movements in very unique circumstances. For the highest level of skill attainment, highly specialized practice is required. In conclusion, maybe the issue of "Generality versus Specificity" should be buried, as both probably operate, in some proportional degree, whenever each "new" activity is attempted and mastered.

Conditions Influencing Transfer

Whenever we discuss the nature of transfer and what can have a transfer effect on what, our thoughts naturally wander to speculations about the ability of people to be good in general in a number of activities. And we ask ourselves to what degree their talents are specialized.

Issues concerning the general capabilities of people to succeed versus the specific nature of task demands were addressed to some degree earlier. The notion of a general motor ability or general athletic ability was refuted. From the previous discussion on transfer, we can see that the ability to perform well in newly-introduced activities depends to a great extent on their relationship to previous experiences, and the extent and quality of these previous experiences.

Furthermore, in complex activities, the general facilitation potential is evidenced primarily *early* in learning. Intensive practice in specific skills and adaptive strategies is a necessity if a high level of proficiency is to be observed. In other words, transfer effects can help at first, but there is no substitution for highly specialized training. And so, when it is stated that someone is an all-round athlete excelling in many sports, it is probable that:

(1) These sports may have elements and demands in common.
(2) Much meaningful, intensive, and specialized training occurred in each activity.

(3) Genetic factors helped influencing potential for body build, temperament, and other personal characteristics.

(4) A high need to achieve was present in regard to each activity.

As we can see, many factors alone or in combination can influence achievement in one or more activities. Since we are concerned here with transfer, it is evident that prior learnings can influence new learnings—in general, but specialization suggests the need for much specific practice in a particular activity (see Figure 8–2).

Besides *situational* and *task relationships*, other conditions should be present if transfer is to occur. Transfer is more likely to happen if under the initial learning conditions there is an *intention* to learn for subsequent potential uses, to apply the learning to future related tasks and circumstances. In addition, *level of learning, or skill*, in a first task, is a important consideration. Greater skill learning leads to greater transfer potential in related tasks. And it is of great importance that the learner realize—*perceive*—the relationship between that which has been experienced and that which is to be experienced.

IMPROVING RETENTION

Retention refers to what we remember, or what we don't forget. In reality, most tests of "learning" are in fact tests of what we retain. And, in reality, considering all the testing situations in school and tests of athletic capabilities in competition, the ability to retain that which has been learned, and produce it in the test context, is what counts.

If you recall, earlier in the material we discussed the sequence of processes of human activities in the learning/performance of acts. At that time, we made

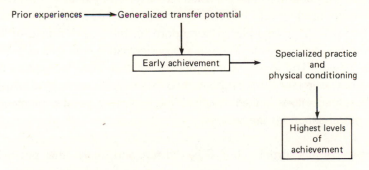

Figure 8–2. Expectations for achievement in a particular activity.

distinctions with regard to short-term memory *(STM)* and long-term memory *(LTM)*. Short-term memory, the working memory, operates in the learning/ performance of all activities. Retention over time, however, is a function of how well information or skill representation was made in long-term memory, and how easily and accurately it can be retrieved. Consequently, any discussion about the improvement of retention must center around conditions, techniques, and processes to improve "putting it in" and "getting it out," where "it" refers to the information of interest.

HOW GENERALIZABLE ARE MEMORY FUNCTIONS?

It is true that memory can be trained to improve through the use of such processes as imagery, coding, chunking, and labeling. In those learning situations in which such memory skills are applicable, their use should facilitate long-term storage.

It is frequently thought that memory is improved in general through experience in certain activities, such as chess playing. It happens that chess players, from grand masters to beginners have been studied quite extensively. Do you think that the expert chess player has and develops more extraordinary visual imagery, a memory quality that encourage success in a number of circumstances? Or is the chess player's talent strictly limited to application to the way the game of chess is typically played?

Consider the following quote from an article in the June 1980 issue of *Science,* written by Larkin, McDermott, Simon, and Simon. It summarizes a typical experiment:

> The subject is shown a position from an actual chess game with about 25 pieces on the board for 5 to 10 seconds, and is then required to reproduce the position from memory. A master or grand master can perform this task with about 90 percent accuracy; a weaker player will do well to replace five or six pieces correctly on the board. Next, the experiment is repeated with 25 pieces placed at random on the board instead of in an arrangement from a game. The expert's performance now falls to the level of the novice. The experiment demonstrates that these perceptual skills stem from no innate general superiority of memory, or capacity to visualize, for the superiority is limited strictly to the expert's area of competence—only typical situations are retained.

Did these results surprise you? They did me, and many other people!

Practice Conditions

The environment in which practice occurs, in which a task is learned, needs to be considered in relation to when and where the task is to be performed in the future. Situational, or *contextual*, cues are learned as well as specific information or skills. It is one thing to put something into *LTM;* another matter to retrieve it. *Retrieval* is best when a test of retention is given within in the same context in which something is learned. There are many experts who feel that once something is placed into *LTM*, it is never really forgotten. It's a matter of getting it out. The right cues (environmental, contextual) would help. In sport, the message is clear: practice a certain amount of time under the conditions that will be present in the forthcoming event.

Retention is also affected by the *meaningfulness* of the learning activities. More meaningful tasks, as perceived by the learner, when practiced during training, will be retained better. Although teachers and coaches think they know what's best for their students and athletes (and they may be right), the learners are the ones who need to be convinced. Cognitions and attitudes must be influenced.

Retention of a task can be influenced negatively by learning prior to or after the learning of that task. (We are dealing with transfer effects.) *Retroactive inhibition* refers to the negative effect of a second-learned task on a first-learned task. *Proactive inhibition* indicates the negative influence of a first-learned task on a second-learned task. In other words, the retention of an activity of interest will be affected by what is experienced prior to and following the learning of that activity. If the highest retention of an activity is of interest, consideration must be given to the kinds of activities experienced prior to and after practice in that activity, and to the relationships between them. There should be a minimum of competing responses; retention will be best when this is the case.

Furthermore, retention is increased when *over-learning* or *over-practice* occurs. In other words, more practice on a task leads to a more permanent learning (retention) of it. Research indicates that more practice leads to better retention, although the results are not necessarily proportional between amount of practice and performance during retention; there is a point of diminishing returns.

In a typical study, practice for one group of subjects would proceed until a criterion is attained. A second group (the fifty per cent group) would retain criterion, and receive fifty per cent more trials. For example, a subject who took twelve trials to reach the criterion would be given six (fifty per cent of twelve) additional trials. Another group might be given 100 per cent more trials after achieving the criterion performance. We could continue with possible groups. What we would probably find is that (1) more practice (additional trials) leads to more retention; and (2) the increments in retentional performance are not proportional to the amount of initial performance—there are diminishing returns for the amount of practice spent.

An additional consideration, the *sequence* (if there is a sequence) of acts learned, might very well determine how well each act is retained. A *primacy-recency* effect is common in tests of retention in *serial learning* (the learning of a sequence of items). In other words, the *order* in which items of equal difficulty are learned are influenced the way they are retained. Typically, in verbal learning, the best remembered items will be the first (primacy) and last (recency) ones; the ones in the middle will be remembered least well. Different reasons have been offered for this phenomenon, but the most reasonable is that there is the least interference in learning for beginning and ending items. Middle items are interfered with by the learning of earlier items (proactive inhibition) and later items (retroactive inhibition).

A test of the serial-position effect was undertaken by Richard Magill and Martha Dowell (1977), using a linear slide apparatus. Blindfolded subjects had to move a handle to a stop position on the apparatus, and learn either three, six, or nine positions. Looking at Figure 8–3, we can observe that with three positions to be recalled, no position effect was observed. But the bowed serial position curve did occur with six and nine positions. The best performance was noted with the first positions, second best was the last positions, while the poorest recall occurred in the middle positions in general.

To summarize, considerations for retention with regard to practice conditions include:

(1) The contextual (situational) relationship of practice and testing.
(2) The perceived meaningfulness of the learning task.
(3) Prior and subsequent experiences with regard to the task of interest.
(4) Amount of practice.
(5) The sequence of learned items.

To improve retention,

(1) Have practice and testing conditions similar, so that contextual cues are available for information retrieval.
(2) Influence the cognitive and affective processes of the learner so that practice conditions and learning tasks are considered meaningful.
(3) Try to insure that activity prior to and after practice on the task of interest will not interfere with the retention task.

(4) Provide sufficient practice, the amount of which will depend on the level of retention desired.

(5) If a sequence of items, materials, or tasks is to be learned, perhaps practice should be such that the order is changed every so often, so as to minimize the order effect (the serial positioning curve, i.e., the primacy-recency effect).

Finally, tests of retention should not be *delayed* too long from the time of last practice. For a more complex task, periods of no practice lead to immediate declines in performance. Refamiliarity with a task and contextual cues, and reactivating appropriate movement patterns in space and in proper timing, usually lead to performance decrements at first on tests of retention when long periods of no practice have preceded them.

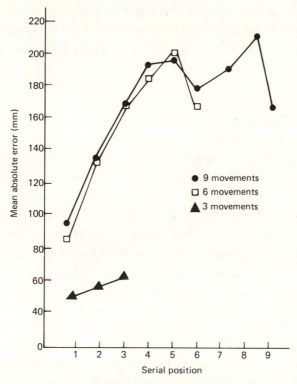

Figure 8–3. Recall as a function of serial position and number of movements. (From R. A. Magill and M. N. Dowell, Serial-position effects in motor short-term memory. *Journal of Motor Behavior,* 1977, 9, 319–324.)

Influencing Memory Processes

Cognitive psychology, the study of the way individuals process information, informs us that many techniques can be used by a person to improve memory; that is, to relocate information from *STM* to *LTM*, and in a organized fashion. Some of the primary techniques, at least with verbal material are:

(1) *Rehearsal.* Sufficient time for internally rehearsing information is necessary if it is to be stored effectively.

(2) *Chunking.* Only a limited amount of information can be processed and stored at one time; chunking it allows more information to be dealt with. For example, instead of trying to memorize each digit of a phone number separately, chunk or clump them in groups of twos and threes or a group of three numbers and a group of four numbers.

(3) *Labeling.* Verbalizing information may help to make it more meaningful, thereby increasing retention potential.

(4) *Coding or mnemonics.* Special ways of categorizing or tagging information may be associated with retention and retrieval. Catch expressions, rhymes, or associations can be made with the information that is to be memorized.

The above and other strategies are effective in learning verbal matter. To the extent that verbal directions or other information have to be learned when acquiring motor skill, these strategies may be useful in the psychomotor domain. These strategies may be applicable to the movement patterns themselves.

There are strategies to consider that are unique to motor skills, mainly those related to kinesthetic information. As we learn written information or information about movement, it is transformed and *coded* in memory. Coding is a process of modifying information so that it can be stored and retrieved more effectively. It is coded for convenience and to enhance the retrieval process; that is, to facilitate memory when that information is needed again. When a movement is "stored" in memory, what type of information can be coded? What types of kinesthetic information are most important for memory effectiveness?

Two types of kinesthetic information have been studied with laboratory tasks: location and distance. Blindfolded subjects have to reposition levers, and their accuracy in this test is determined. They could rely on location cues, distance cues, or both. It has been well established that location cues can be retained and rehearsed in memory. Diewert and Roy (1978) have found that memory of movement-extent information can benefit from either a location strategy or a counting strategy. They suggest that there is flexibility in the way movement-extent information is coded.

Memory depends on the availability of processing capacity for a location strategy, but capacity is not so important for a counting strategy. Diewert and Roy concluded that kinesthetic information is not useful for extent (distance) memory; instead, coding strategies are more beneficial. They speculated that locations may be coded and retained more accurately than extent, which may be due to less processing complexity than that associated with location coding.

Types of Tasks

Generally speaking, motor skills are retained longer than verbal materials. The often-cited example of riding a bicycle illustrates the point very well. Once you have learned to ride a bike, or swim, you will be able to perform these activities even without many years of practice in them. Gross motor activities can be retained for a long long time. Take a look, if you will, at Figure 8–4. Judith Meyers (1967) tested five groups of high school girls with different lengths of lay-offs (nonperformance) following the learning of a balance task. When the groups were retested, after delays of ten minutes, one day, one week, four weeks, and thirteen weeks, respectively, no significant loss in retention was observed. However, activities that require a great deal of precision in their execution will obviously not be retained as well without regular practice.

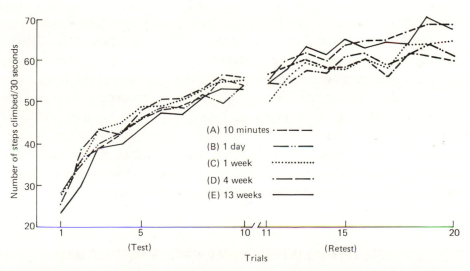

Figure 8–4. Mean performance scores for each of the five retention groups. (From J. L. Meyers, Retention of balance coordination learning as influenced by extended lay-offs. *Research Quarterly,* 1967, 38, 72–78.)

The two major reasons offered for the longer-term retention of motor skills in general than of verbal material are (1) *Over-practice*, and (2) *Lack of interfering intervening activities*. Many motor skills are practiced proportionally longer than verbal materials are studied. In addition, we acquire so much verbal information in our lifetime, much of which may compete with other information. As to motor skills, we don't learn that many, and most of them are quite unique. Thus, there is less of a chance that interference will occur between experiences in various motor skills.

The Loss in Retention

Typically, performance decrements after a period of no practice have been attributed to:

(1) Decay or disuse
(2) Activity interference
(3) Problems with retrieval from memory

Simply not practicing an act of some degree of difficulty will usually result in performance decrements at a later date. This concept has been called *decay theory*, or *the theory of disuse*. By not "using" response patterns in particular situations, the ability to respond correctly will "decay." However, perhaps more important than the time delay between the last practice and the next attempt is what happens during that interval. If activities experienced will compete (*negative interference* or transfer) with a prior learning, retention of the latter will be lowered. When studying for a written test to be given the next day, should we rest or sleep as much as possible between the study period and testing period, or is it all right to read other written matter and participate in activities during this period? On this latter problem, Figure 8–5 illustrates data showing the comparison of various intervals of sleeping and activity between two testing periods. Evidently, inactivity yields more effective results, for no competing responses interfere with the retention of the matter under this condition. An increase in waking hours results in a decline in performance.

STUDYING WHAT INFLUENCES RETENTION

We could analyze disuse theory and interference theory as to which is a more correct interpretation of what influences retention, in the following manner.

Suppose we had four groups of subjects, randomly selected and placed into groups. They all might learn a task to some criterion. One day (twenty-four hours) later they are to be tested for retention.

Each group would be treated differently during the twenty-four hour interval. One group might be asked to rest and, if active, do things completely unrelated to the task. Groups 2, 3, and 4 would be given activities to undertake, related to the criterion-learned task. However, the amount of time for this purpose would differ from group to group. The design of the experiment would look like this:

Groups	Test	Intervening Activity	Retention
1	X	None	X
2	X	2 hours	X
3	X	4 hours	X
4	X	8 hours	X

Most likely, achievement in the retention test would be in the order as presented above. A difference in retention is apparently due to what occurs during the intervening period, from the learning test to the retention test, not merely to the passage of time.

Finally, as was mentioned before, retention may be impaired due to an inability to *retrieve* from memory the right response in a particular situation. If information is stored in a certain situation context, and if in a test of retention the same situational context exists, possibilities are much greater that retention performance will be improved.

Reminiscence

A phenomenon termed *reminiscence* has been observed on some occasions in tests of retention. It refers to an *improvement* in performance in a test of retention as compared to the last previous score or scores, and is due to inactivity in the task. Why should this occur?

Most often the reminiscence effect is due to artificially depressed prior practice scores. For instance, such is the case during massed practice. With continuous practices of the task, performance begins to worsen due to boredom or fatigue. A rest from the activity will allow the person to demonstrate a truer

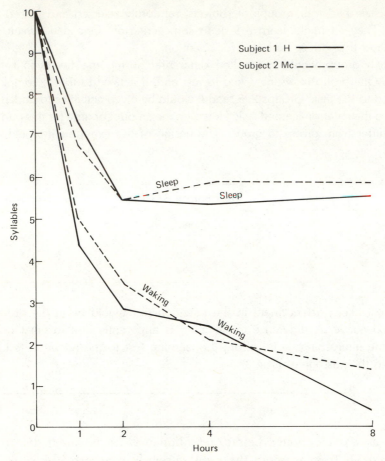

Figure 8–5. Retention as a function of various time intervals of sleep and waking. There is an observed marked difference on the rate of forgetting during sleeping and waking. (From J. G. Jenkins and K. M. Dallenbach, Oblivescence during sleep and waking. *American Journal of Psychology*, 1924, 35, 605–612.)

(probably higher) level of achievement when he or she returns to the activity. Likewise, what is probably called "staleness" in sport—a condition associated with lower levels of achievement after a reasonable success—may be relieved after a rest period or participation in other activities. Continuous repetition of an act can take its toll.

Do you play golf? Have you ever experienced reasonable progress with your shots and scores, and then everything seems to "fall apart"? The scores and shots worsen. Then you laid off for a few months or so. Upon resuming playing golf, your shots and scores were much better than when you stopped. Perhaps you were much more relaxed. You expected less of yourself. There are times when "a break in the action" can work to a person's advantage.

SUMMARY

As we have seen, there are many ways to influence the learner directly in task-learning situations. On one hand, the practice environment and conditions can be constructed favorably. On the other hand, learner processes involved in learning can be analyzed carefully and ways to affect them positively applied.

Motivation was analyzed in terms of conditional effects; that is, the role of rewards as an external means in directing behavior. It was also analyzed with a perspective toward personal cognitive processes that are activated when intrinsic motivation is present. Locus of control (internal) when undertaking an activity, and type of attributions (like effort) made following performance, can apparently influence achievement in a positive manner. Control and perceived causative factors can be modified through external guidance, if that is desirable. Both intrinsic and extrinsic sources of motivation can influence activity preference and persistence in practice, but intrinsic forces are generally the more advantageous of the two. Achievement motivation principles serve as guidelines to realize high and specific goals; and these principles represent a blueprint to success.

Feedback must be present if learning is to occur. Many times feedback is insufficient or else not attended to properly, thereby creating the need for supplementary feedback (knowledge of results). Consideration must be given to the feedback—whether it is concurrent or terminal feedback; if terminal, whether it is immediate or delayed; the nature of the feedback—from what sources it comes; and the extent of the feedback. When discussing transfer, it was stressed that all previous learning influences present learning; that it is rare that we really learn something completely new after eight years of age. The degree of relationship between the present and the past, as to stimuli and responses, will account for a good degree of potential for positive or negative transfer. Most likely, positive transfer from the past is of more importance in a general way as "new" skills are being learned. Facilitative effects, in other words, are early and general. However, for high degrees of skill in complex tasks, much task-specific practice must occur. Refinement and synchronization of acts do not depend on generalized transfer functions but rather on practice of those skills in the appropriate performance context.

Finally, retention was addressed. That which is remembered is dependent upon situational arrangements during practice and the appropriate use of personal control processes during learning to influence long-term memory. Practice conditions that promote overlearning influence retention greatly. Such memory processes as chunking, labeling, and coding put information into LTM in an organized manner and make it easier to access it. Retention is improved when tasks are meaningful—as perceived by the learner. Two leading conceptual orientations to describe retention potential have to do with decay (loss of memory from lack of use over time) and inhibition (owing to competing responses—more recent learnings, if related, will interfere with the retention of previous learnings).

All in all, it was demonstrated that learning and achievement need not be a haphazard process. Systematic plans to improve the arrangement of practice environments and conditions, as well as the functioning of personal processes, will lead to the most favorable results.

REFERENCES AND SUGGESTED READINGS

Covington, M. V. and Beery, R. G. *Self-worth and school learning.* New York: Holt, Rinehart and Winston, 1976.

Deci, E. L. *Intrinsic motivation.* New York: Plenum Press, 1975.

Dickinson, J. *A behavioral analysis of sport.* Princeton, New Jersey: Princeton Book Co., 1977.

Diewert, G. L. and Roy, E. A. Coding strategy for memory of movement extent information. *Journal of Experimental Psychology: Human Learning and Memory,* 1978, 4, 666–675.

Ellis, H. C. *The transfer of learning.* New York: Macmillan Publishing Co., Inc., 1965.

Klatzsky, R. L. *Human memory: structures and processes.* San Francisco, W. H. Freeman, 1980.

Magill, R. A. and Dowell, M. N. Serial-position effects in motor short-term memory. *Journal of Motor Behavior,* 1977, 9, 319–323.

Norman, D. A. *Memory and attention.* New York: John Wiley, 1976.

Wallace, S. A. and Hagler, R. W. Knowledge of performance and the learning of a closed motor skill. *Research Quarterly,* 1979, 50, 265–271.

Weiner, B. (ed.) *Achievement motivation and attribution theory.* Morristown, New Jersey: General Learning Press, 1974.

Weiner, B. The role of affect in rational (attributional) approaches to human motivation. *Educational Researcher,* 1980, 9, 4–11.

9

THE

HIGHLY

SKILLED

So far it has been shown that many personal processes and various learning conditions can influence the acquisition of skill. But for a learner to be really skilled in an activity implies that these processes are operational in the most desirable manner. Of course, the realization of a high skill level is dependent on many other factors as well.

As complex as many motor skills are and as the demands placed on the performers are, it is little wonder that the combination of so many general and specific factors can lead to successful performances. In any sport, nutrition, health, body build, and conditioning are each important considerations. Likewise, the knowledge of and the ability to executive specific skills and tactics in the context of competition are necessary prerequisites for achievement.

In addition, the strategies that the learner uses can influence performance. Cognitive processes may act in many ways. In sports situations, for example, "mental orientation" and decisions are associated with training in preparation for competition, readying just before the contest, directing activities during the contest, and interpreting and adjusting to the outcome of competition. Effective strategies are those that improve the way processes work. As we will see, one of the major differences between the highly skilled and the less skilled is the type of strategies used by each in the same situation.

Assuming that we never come close to tapping our capacity limits for achievement in any activity, we need to learn how to improve the operation of processes that can lead to the realization and maintenance of skill. Strategies that seem to be closely allied with skilled performances will be analyzed in this chapter. The automation of skill is an important concept that needs to be addressed. So is the notion of the adaptability of behaviors. We will also focus our attention on how highly adept people control and direct specific, brief movements or a sequential series of acts. The chapter will conclude with some special considerations with regard to the nature of strategies.

WHAT DOES IT MEAN TO BE SKILLED?

As has been suggested earlier in this book, skill is a function of many interacting factors. It refers to one's ability to perform objectives according to high and specifically-stated standards. Saying it simply, skill involves "doing the right thing at the right time."

Depending on what's required in a movement or a series of movements— accuracy, speed, adaptability, form, energy conservation, etc.—movements meet situational demands. And the more skilled someone is, the greater the probability of overcoming more stressful and demanding circumstances. Specialized training

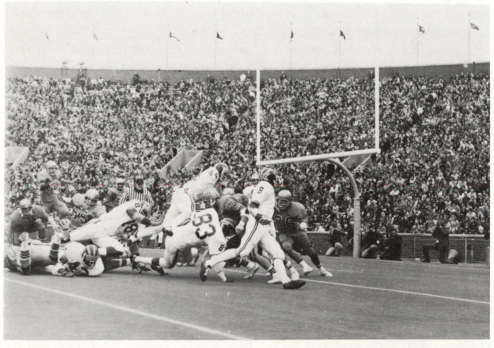

Featherkill Studios, Burnsville, MN

Performance strategies for all football players must work well and quickly if a play is to succeed.

leads to the refinement of the attributes necessary to achieve in a particular task. One learns techniques to influence actions—by controlling and appropriately directing thought processes and emotions. The ability to self-control and self-regulate, and to be able to do this consistently, is the mark of highly proficient performers.

Some motor activities demand quick decisions and fast responses. The performance of the best achievers appear to be automatic, to be programmed. Other activities require adaptive and flexible responses as situations change suddenly, often unpredictably. And yet within other activities, both automatic and adaptive behaviors may be needed, again depending on circumstances. The highly skilled in a specific activity can make the appropriate decisions and initiate more or less consciously planned movements to meet the requirements of each situation.

WHAT IS STRATEGY?

An effective *strategy* has been described as the simplest and most efficient means of processing the information inherent in a situation. A strategy is a skill of self-management that the learner acquires to govern the processes of attending, learning, and thinking; it governs behavior. By using a strategy, a learner imposes some type of structure on cue and movement information so that an act or information is learned and retrieved more effectively. He or she makes an association of what works in a particular situation.

Some generalizations can be made about strategies. For instance, strategies characteristically: (1) involve systematic analysis and processing; (2) require repeated attempts at a solution; and (3) involve the development of rules, to be applied to the same or similar situations.

An instructional strategy that is imposed by the instructor on the learner may be designed to help the learner to acquire a skill as quickly as possible, or to facilitate transfer effectiveness or problem-solving in the future. While some imposed strategies may increase the rate of initial skill acquisition, they may not facilitate learning in transfer situations where no instructor is present. In the latter case, this can only be achieved when a learner becomes capable of self-generating strategies, whether they have been initially externally directed or self-generated.

With a self-initiated strategy, the learner is capable of determining a procedure that is compatible with his or her personal cognitive capabilities and cognitive style for the learning of a task or a category of related tasks. Strategy choice is partially determined by the particular situation so a sound procedure would appear to be to instruct learners initially in the use of learning strategies if they are ignorant about them. Once a learner comprehends the nature of and the reasons for the use of particular strategies for the acquisition of skill, he or she should be capable of self-generating strategies in related future learning environments. Through a feeling of self-control and self-direction, decision making is improved and self-initiated.

THE ROLE OF STRATEGIES AND COGNITIVE PROCESSES

Students in typical classroom situations and athletes in conventional training programs have experiences that emphasize teaching and coaching methods. *Sport-specific* knowledge, skills, and tactics must be acquired; but so must *supportive learnings.* The ability to problem-solve, adapt, accommodate, and in general to apply strategies to expected and unexpected situations provides the athlete with more comprehensive tools to train and to compete favorably. Other supportive learnings include the ability to analyze oneself in terms of dispositional and readiness states to learn/perform, and what to do (self-management skills) about the presence of inappropriate states. The relationship of these considerations to achievement is diagrammed in Figure 9–1.

Whereas the sport-specific learnings of the athlete are typically managed under the direction of a coach, supportive learnings are not. The same is true in classroom settings. Supportive learnings are taken for granted. They are neglected.

Cognitive (mental) processes are involved in the learning and performance of motor skills to a greater extent than is usually realized. Superior performers maximize the involvement *or* detachment of such processes before, during, and after learning/performance. Better strategies should enhance the selection and processing of information, as well as decision-making. In other words, the highly skilled are highly skilled in part due to their ability to use strategies appropriate for each situation.

Some form of control can be potentially exerted by the learner/performer from the time information enters his or her system until it is transformed and responded to in the form of movement activity. The control may be continually active (conscious) during the activity. It may be preplanned, in which case the activity proceeds as if subconsciously undertaken. Or a switching mechanism may operate, alternating back and forth from conscious to subconscious control.

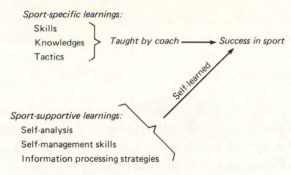

Figure 9–1. Learnings that contribute to potential to achieve in a sport.

The better performer learns how to control acts. One of the primary differences between the highly skilled and the less skilled is the degree and type of conscious involvement prior to, during, and following motor performance. Conscious planning, focus, and/or intervention at a particular point in the execution of acts must be determined according to task demands. The capabilities of the person will be reflected accordingly.

Control processes, according to Geoffrey Underwood (1978), are "those processes that are not permanent features of memory, but are instead transient phenomena under the control of the subject [person] . . ." (p. 237)." Many internal operations can occur. The choice of the right ones as applied in the appropriate situations will make the difference in performance outcomes.

However, the person does not totally influence any situation, nor does the reverse probably happen. Whereas behaviorists might lead us to view human behavior as passively controlled by situational dictates, cognitive psychologists suggest that people actively control their environments. The truth probably lies somewhere in the middle. Behaviors are not produced without cues or stimuli, and these behaviors are directed by them. But all people do not respond similarly to the same events, thereby demonstrating some degree of self-determination. In a sense, then, associated behaviors are indeed developed, but in a person's own way.

The effective operation of a particular control process for a given activity reduces the amount of information that must be selected and transmitted through the human system. Accuracy is truer and processing quicker than otherwise. Processes should be facilitated by the person's activity and use of pertinent strategies.

The learning experience is governed by the use of strategies, which in turn activate conscious and, perhaps subsequently, subconscious processes. The relationships hypothesized would be that situations activate particular strategies that influence cognitive processes in this way:

(1) A situation activates potential *alternative strategies.*

(2) A particular *appropriate strategy* influences a corresponding *cognitive process.*

(3) Situation⟶ Strategy⟶ Process

The learning of a motor skill or a verbal skill reflects a problem that must be solved. The behaviors involved in acquiring both types of skill are very similar, in that the learner must identify and interpret the problem, utilize strategies to facilitate the processing of information so that he or she can devise a plan that will lead to possible solutions, produce those solutions, and then decide which is the best solution. An example would be learning to make the right kind of tennis serve to the right place against an opponent. His or her strengths and weaknesses must be analyzed so that the weaknesses can be exploited.

Self-management strategies allow information processing strategies to operate more effectively. They have to do with establishing right attitudes (a readiness) toward learning and performance, coping with concentration deficits, dealing with potential anxiety, and in general, being able to monitor progress and personal state.

Both information processing and self-management strategies reflect potential cognitive control over performances and feelings. When individuals possess a larger variety of effective strategies that can satisfy situational demands and personal needs, their achievements should be much greater.

THE STATE OF READINESS

Readiness to learn and perform can be defined as the student's or athlete's willingness, receptivity, or desire to acquire information and skills, or in general to perform well. Several factors that may influence psychological preparatory and maitenance states are:

1. prior experience, familiarity, and skill level in relation to present activities.

2. previous successes.

3. cognitive style (i.e., personal approaches to the solution of problems), and

4. attitudes toward and in the situation.

The unique combination of many factors at any given time results in the person's attitudinal, arousal, attentional, and cognitive state at that moment.

Both cognitive and affective factors influence the learning of motor skills. It is difficult to deal with cognitive and affective factors separately, observe Spielberger, Gonzalez, and Fletcher (1978), since the two are closely interrelated. Athletes as well as any other people involved with gross motor skills must be psychologically, physically, and intellectually ready to learn, retain, and perform. They need to be able to identify their dispositional states to perform, through the application of pertinent self-evaluation strategies. Conflict between the ideal and the less than ideal needs to be resolved. Analytical training, with an understanding of what to do about particular problems, writes R. B. Stuart (1977), should facilitate the effectiveness of athletes in a variety of circumstances. With or without training, the highly skilled seem to possess a great ability to self-evaluate and to take any appropriate steps to resolve internal conflict.

Many attempts are being made in the sports world to help athletes, or help athletes to help themselves, to attain readiness to train and to compete. Optimal states of attention, concentration, motivation, relaxation, anxiety, and the like need to be determined. As is the case with the learning or performance of specific skills, learning how to be prepared, oriented, or ready for competition is a major factor in the determination of performance outcome. There is much yet to be known about general dispositional states, about the unique concerns for individuals with unique characteristics, and about how to help people become more effective as to the way they attempt to acquire knowledge and skill, to retain them, and to cope with situations that appear to be new but are related to others previously experienced.

While instructions, or orienting tasks, may be able to influence learning positively to some degree, little learning and poor performance will occur if a person is not psychologically prepared to achieve. Self-analysis strategies make possible the personal determination of psychological readiness, and should influence decisions to undertake responsibilities and how to proceed. The readiness of the learner not only influences the initial motivation toward the task, but

STRATEGIES FOR READYING ONESELF FOR ATHLETIC COMPETITION

Although there might be agreement as to certain strategies that might operate effectively for most people in the same situation, there are instances where there is disagreement. In fact, different approaches might suit different types of people very well. Consider the following description from *Newsweek* of the way two outstanding baseball players "do their thing":

If George Brett were to write a how-to book on hitting, it might go something like this. First tip: never think about the game ahead of time. Get to the ball park early, so you can work on your superstitutions. "The other day I couldn't find my lucky T shirt. I panicked." When the game starts, notice who's pitching, but don't think about what he'll throw; it doesn't matter. Step into the batter's box and blank out everything. And, oh yes, When you're standing on first—or second or third—take off your good-luck sweatband. Such is the uncerebral approach to baseball of the man who is threatening to become the first .400 hitter in 39 years.

Pitcher Steve Stone's instructional guide would be a very different matter. Always think about the game ahead of time. Take the phone off the hook. Lie down on your bed, close your eyes. Then pitch the entire game-to-be in your head, getting out every batter at least four times, plus a couple of pinch hitters. Don't stop until you can envision pitching coach Ray Miller congratulating you on a complete game. The beauty of this approach, as Stone can attest, is that it helps turn a lifetime .500 pitcher into a crafty twenty-game winner. "I'm a good pitcher," says the Baltimore right-hander, who won No. 20 last week, "but not a great one. So I have to outsmart the opposition. If I go on instinct, I go to the shower."

("A Phenomenal Odd Couple," *Newsweek,* Sept. 1, 1980, p. 80.)

These contrasting approaches have been remarkably successful for each baseball player. They suggest why it is impossible to force each person into the same mold. Often we try out different strategies, and use what works best for us.

---

the manner in which motivation is maintained during learning and performance as well. For example, an athlete enters a situation that requires the acquisition of a new skill. If he or she has had limited background experience with similar skills, and does not know how to determine personal readiness for learning, the situation could prove to be anxiety-provoking, and the level of arousal may become much more intense than is required for that task.

On the other hand, if the same athlete had learned self-evaluation, anxiety-reduction, and coping strategies, the preparatory state would have been recognized, excessive arousal levels would have been reduced, and performance would proceed as hoped (e.g., Nideffer, 1976; Wenz and Strong, 1980). Another possibility is that the learner would determine his or her readiness state as presently unfit for the task, and would withdraw from the situation until remedial procedures could be invoked. Then he or she would return to the situation, ready to achieve. Those who are skilled in the mechanical aspects of a movement can be even more skilled when they learn how to ready themselves for performance and to maintain an ideal psychological state during performance.

PROCESSING INFORMATION

The stages in the processing of information do not operate equally effectively in people with different levels of skill in a particular activity. To filter appropriate cues while simultaneously blocking irrelevant information is difficult for the less skilled individual. In fact, this may be one of the reasons he or she is less skilled. In contrast, the better performer is able to abstract the commonality among inputs and employ an effective strategy for the recognition and selection of information.

In addition, the beginner may be unaware of how to use the appropriate control processes for the transmission of information through the various processing mechanisms, while the advanced performer knows when and where to activate certain cognitive processes, and when to have them operate at a subconscious or what appears to be an automatic level. The varying skill level demonstrated by beginners and highly proficient performers may be accounted for in part by their different abilities to use strategies appropriately to process information, as was mentioned earlier.

The major point is that many people have similar capacities to process information, but some—the best performers—probably process much more expediently. They use their capacities to fullest advantage. Through experience, we can store much information and learn to recognize what to do in the present situation. We retrieve what is necessary upon recognition of familiar cues. "The accumulation of experience may allow people to behave in ways that are very nearly optimal in situations to which their experience is pertinent, but will be of little help when genuinely novel situations are presented" (Simon, 1978, p. 503). Furthermore as Simon points out, "Direct retrieval of possible courses of action as a result of recognizing familiar features of the problem situation provides a major (one might almost say *the* major) basis for professional performance in complex problem situations" (p. 504). This, of course, is true in a specific sport, assuming the person possesses the appropriate movement skills.

It is important to use advantageously self-management skills related to readiness to learn/perform, anticipation, emotional control, concentration, stimulus recognition, selective attention, the use of channel capacity, the retrieval of related information for later use, the planning and selecting of a motor program (plans) for present use, the organization of behaviors, the utilization of response-produced feedback, and other such self-help processes. Performance is improved with the utilization of appropriate strategies with regard to these considerations.

This point has been established from a variety of research perspectives. Differences have been noted in strategy use by expert and novice subjects in solving physics problems. Also, chess players with different skill levels have been differentiated for a number of cognitive factors, such as experience and the ability to formulate principles and plans relative to situations on the chess board (Hearst and Wierzbicki, 1979). Furthermore, W. T. Gallwey (1976) helped to introduce Eastern world concepts to tennis. Those strategies apparently developed in world class performers were emphasized for beginners; e.g., imaging, concentrating, relaxing, and in general "letting the body do its thing." The importance of recognizing the role of cognitive processes and information-processing capabilities in the acquisition and maintenance of skill is gaining increased attention from experimental psychologists, industrial psychologists, educators, military trainers, and sport psychologists.

IMPROVING THE OPERATION OF INTERNAL MECHANISMS

Let us take a moment to return to some fundamental information processing considerations: the use of long-term memory (LTM) and short-term memory (STM), the nature of attention, and the role of feedback. But here we will see how the highly skilled differ from the less skilled in the strategies they use to enhance information processing operations.

Using Long-Term Memory

Beginners lack experience, and thereby lack a proper reference system for recognizing and judging new situations as being similar to previous situations. Thus, less skilled performers are unable to activate the desired memory representations, because the memory isn't there. They also process information at a slower rate.

Speed of information retrieval from the LTM is a crucial area of difference between skill levels. With more experience, more situations are encountered, and these tend to be recognized when they recur. Similarities between stimuli affect memory access time, and since advanced performers can categorize more situations as similar, and yet make just-noticeable distinctions if necessary, they can activate the proper memory representations to anticipate future incoming stimuli. Additionally, the differences in strategy use between advanced and novice performers at the time the information was originally stored leads to variations in their LTM access and retrieval times. Thus, experience is one factor that can be used to explain differences in LTM functioning, as experience is probably the major causal element in the determination of what information is to be attended to and recognized.

The Functioning of Short-term Memory

It is in the short-term memory mechanism that most of the information transformations are active. Additionally, most of the processing differences among individuals can be identified as occurring in the STM. The performance variability that may be noted both between and within individuals is often due to the differential use and effectiveness of their strategies for the organization of information.

When learners are at the same developmental stage, variations in processing abilities have been speculated by Chi (1976) not to be due to differences in structural capacity. Rather, these differences occur in the functional utilization of the short-term memory; that is, the strategies a learner uses to process information. The divergence in performance that is evidenced between high- and low-skilled learners is due in part to strategy use. Better (more adaptable) learners are more capable of shifting from an old, less efficient strategy to a new, more appropriate strategy during the course of skill acquisition.

Highly-skilled individuals are more likely to invoke a unique or perhaps a modified strategy as new items are entered into the STM. The improved coding of information at the time of storage enables advanced learners to evidence superior performances at the time of testing. This is very similar to the notion that elaborate or enriched coding (the transformation of information within the human processing system) during storage will lead to better performance at a later date. Since encoding usually refers to information reduction, elaboration, modification, or reconstruction (see Hall, 1978, for a review) and probably influences what is stored in memory, the types of strategy used will be of great influence.

Performance differences may very well be due in large part to variability in strategy use between people as to their processing of information in the STM. Performance differences between high- and low-skilled individuals on certain memory tasks, e.g., digit span, have been found to be due to the use of different strategies. The same conclusions have been reached with a limb positioning motor short-term memory task. Consequently, the ability of a learner to devise and implement appropriate strategies for handling information apparently determines the level of his or her subsequent performance on both verbal and motor short-term memory tasks.

Housner and Hoffman (1978) showed that high-visual imagers were able to reproduce limb position end locations better than low-visual imagers. The movement reproduction superiority of the former was evidenced over retention intervals that included either an interfering activity or a task rehearsal activity (imaging). The consistent results across all conditions were attributed to differences in the ability of the two groups to utilize the designated strategy of imaging.

It is clear that strategy use in short-term memory is one determinant of short-term memory performance, whether the task is verbal or motoric in nature. The greater ability of highly-skilled individuals to process, manipulate, and organize information in this mechanism leads to a more appropriate and efficient performance. This is most evident when motor skills are investigated, as performers must quickly process information and decide on which movements must be made, in what direction, and with what speed. Greater organizational characteristics can be attributed to the strategies of highly-skilled individuals (Gentile and Nacson, 1976) that enable these persons to encode all the necessary information at the time of storage. Consequently, most or all potential retrieval cues would also be stored, and this should lead to superior performance on a later test.

While advanced performers are able to move efficiently with a minimum expenditure of effort, beginners tend to move in a less efficient manner. After consideration is given to differences in physical capabilities and mechanical techniques, performance differences result from the ability of the highly skilled to form a base of well-organized information in the STM through the use of appropriate rehearsal strategies, and then to select the appropriate motor program.

It should be pointed out that many interactive processes go on between the STM and the LTM. Expectations of success are dependent on previous successes and failures in similar situations. The level of expectation and other motivational factors will bear on the kind of processing that goes on in the STM. Stressors present and individual reactions to them in the form of nonadaptable or coping strategies will also affect processing effectiveness. In other words, there are many intangibles that can help to facilitate or impede strategy selection and execution with regard to processing control. In turn, strategies are needed to make these intangibles work on behalf of the person. It would appear that the highly-skilled performer, in contrast to the less skilled, uses more effective strategies in controlling and directing emotions, reacting to stressors, and in general, maintaining the appropriate arousal level for the task demands. Further, the expectations in performance level of the former are set reasonably high but realistically.

Attention

Selective attention processes vary among individuals. Individuals differ in their ability to divide or switch attention between competing task demands, and it is probably true that skilled performers possess a better repertoire of strategies for attention than do unskilled performers. A skilled performer is capable of choosing the stimuli that convey the most information while disregarding those stimuli that are of little import or that serve as noise to the system. Unskilled performers, on the other hand, tend to concentrate on both relevant and irrelevant stimuli, thereby overloading their channel capacity. In essence,

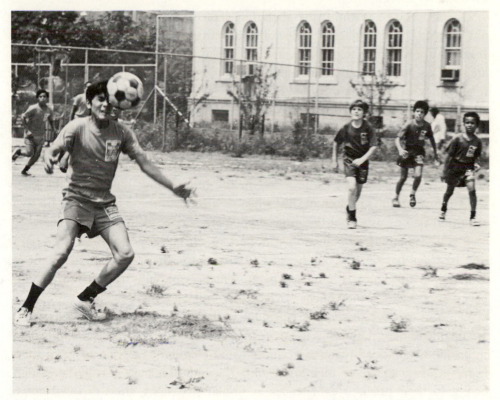

District of Columbia Recreation Department

Concentration is an important skill that needs to be learned.

mature non-skilled performers respond similarly to children who behave in an overinclusive manner (attending to too much information) with respect to selective attention processes. In other words, they take in more information than is needed to execute the task correctly. With age and experience, attention processes improve.

Skilled performers do not behave in an overinclusive manner, and therefore they allocate less of their channel capacity to the task. This leads to an availability of spare capacity that allows these persons to process more information and possibly to engage in parallel processing, e.g., do two tasks simultaneously, anticipate and form potential programs as the activity progresses. This ability is even more pronounced when the learner becomes familiar with the material so that the selective attention and encoding processes do not demand conscious attention.

In contrast, the less skilled individual does not have any spare capacity available and must attend to information in a serial manner. Serial processing is more time-consuming than parallel processing, and thus the speed of a performance is reduced. Adequacy of performance in terms of other criteria may be diminished as well.

Performance dissimilarities between skilled and unskilled individuals are also due to the ability of the highly skilled to extract a large amount of information from a minimal number of cues in the display, whereas less skilled individuals are limited in the amount of information they can transmit. Moreover, the inequalities can also be attributed to the differential use of strategies between the two categories of performers. Whiting (1972) has stated that the information attended to by the skilled performer probably differs from that attended to by the unskilled person. The advanced performer focuses on a critical area of the display and is prepared to perceive particular information quickly and accurately. Inexperienced performers, on the other hand, do not usually know what information is important, nor when to attend to it. They tend to fix their attention on one aspect of the display while other relevant data may be ignored.

This apparent ignorance on the part of unskilled performers is probably due to their having few or no expectations as to what information might be available in the immediate environment. This is especially true with externally-paced tasks, where individuals have to respond to situational dictates, which often occur in a non-predictable way. Due to their inexperience, unskilled persons are unable to determine what to ignore of the contextual display so that pertinent information may be processed accurately and efficiently. Advanced performers, however, are capable of monitoring only the important aspects of the display, owing to their previous experiences in similar situations, their expectations of the information that should be available, and their anticipation of what they must do when this information becomes available. So it is with skilled football quarterbacks in dynamic situations.

The ability to correctly anticipate the arrival of input cues speeds up the perceptual process. The differential and more effective use of selective attention strategies of skilled performers when compared to novices is probably one explanation of divergent performances. Skilled individuals are able to vary their attention systematically, depending on task demands. Certain skills, such as driving a car, require a broad focus of attention, while other tasks, such as hitting a pitched baseball, demand a narrow focus of attention. It is the skilled performer who is capable of increasing or decreasing the width of his or her attentional range as dictated by the situation. The result of these advanced strategic selective attention control processes is that only pertinent information is perceived.

Feedback

Of concern in feedback, information available to the person as a result of his/her actions, are the receptors in the muscles, tendons, and ligaments associated with particular limbs that are responsible for carrying out movement commands. If the commands are accurate and precise, then the effectors simply execute the movement. If the commands are incorrect in any aspect, then the observable performance will be inappropriate. Considering the two possible errors that a performer may make, selection and execution, the effectors are most responsible for correcting errors in response execution.

The correction of response execution errors by the effectors can be carried out through reflexive control within the muscle spindle. Gamma fibers within the spindle receive information that the sequence of muscular contractions is not proceeding according to plan. The gamma system, then, reflexively excites or inhibits the specific motor neuron that controls the extrafusal fibers responsible for the contraction. In this way, execution errors, and even the slightest mismatch between input and output, are corrected and control of the movement can revert to the motor program so that the movement can be completed as planned.

The correction of response execution errors will occur more rapidly in advanced performers than in less-skilled individuals. The extensive amount of practice and the continuous adaptation of strategies necessary to achieve a high level of skill must repeatedly involve successful operation of control processes and of the muscles necessary to perform a movement in an efficient manner. The gamma system of the advanced performer should be more highly tuned to detect and to correct response execution errors than the same system in a novice, because the cortical (highest brain) centers have planned the movement more effectively. Thus, at all levels of skill, there is a system to ensure that the movement is being carried out as planned, and this system is more highly developed in the advanced performer.

Until now, the discussion on effector control has centered around the gamma system, a subconscious form of movement regulation. Obviously, effectors also transmit proprioceptive information for conscious recognition and control on many occasions. This information is recycled throughout the system, to be used immediately and/or as an additional input to the knowledge representation base in LTM. Such is the case with visual feedback or other forms of response-produced information.

If the task or situation is altered due to performance, the input cues change as well. Feedback information can come from the situation or from within the person, but if sources are to be consciously attended to, they must be processed through the set of subsystems already explained. Strategies for the use of feedback are important, as the advanced skilled performer seems to learn which feedback to pay attention to, and when. Once the act is completed, this information should be stored as a reference base for subsequent activity, and beginners need to learn organizational strategies to "catalog" such information correctly in storage, to be retrieved when needed. During an activity, feedback information may be abundant, redundant, or relatively absent. Attention to feedback varies between learners.

CENTRAL AND PERIPHERAL CONTROL FACTORS

The decision-making or response-selection process represents differences in skill levels in two ways. The more advanced performers have greater control over their movements. They evidence shorter latencies (time delays) in the selection process, and they also engage in less error-correcting behavior than their less-skilled counterparts.

Shorter response-selection latencies are the result of greater successful experiences with a particular situation or movement. Extensive practice of a skill often leads to that action becoming programmed, as in *ballistic* (brief and swift) movements where speed is important. A movement under *programmed* (central) *control* can be executed with greater rapidity than a movement under peripheral control. *Peripheral control,* which is most often evidenced by unskilled performers even in ballistic-type movements, is dependent upon *feedback* for effective completion. Since movements under feedback control require more time to execute than programmed movements, unskilled performers respond more slowly. When a tennis shot is hit to them, for example, they will have to think about whether to use a forehand or backhand stance and grip to return it. The skilled player will make the same decision literally without thinking. While this delay in execution may not lead to performance errors during the initial phase of a motor action, it is highly probably that later aspects of a movement will be either error-filled or not performed at all. This would be due to the unskilled performer being unable to prepare the system to accept the new incoming stimuli for which responses must be formulated.

Of course, a truly programmed (or preprogrammed) response is not always desirable. It implies a degree of automaticity, of subconscious control. A reaction to the wrong cue, when under central control, cannot be changed by conscious intervention until at least .20 to .30 of a second has elapsed. The peripheral control of movement suggests a slower movement that is amenable to ongoing modifications and adjustments. It might be suggested that the higher-skilled performer has learned how to adapt, like a thermostat, to response demands. Sometimes movement will be placed under central control, other times under peripheral control.

Realizing their personal limitations, the highly skilled will use movements deliberately under peripheral control in certain situations. When movements do not require speed, then both lower- and higher-skilled performers will rely on peripheral feedback for information. However, the strategies used by the highly skilled as to the monitoring of peripheral (i.e., propioceptive) information differ from those used by lesser-skilled. In the former case, a degree of attention to such information is focused as there is a need, but in the latter case, there probably is more attention given to too much information or else to the less pertinent information. Thus, less-skilled performers would have difficulty successfully completing tasks that demand fast and accurate responses.

Responses that must be formulated and enacted with great accuracy and speed need to be well learned, and therefore can come under program control. As the result of extensive practice, the skilled performer establishes a repertoire of programmable movement subroutines and action plans that can be performed without much conscious attention. These subroutines are controlled at a lower level, which frees the system to attend to other relevant situational inputs.

A Hybrid System

D. Glencross (1977) substantiated this point by stating that the higher centers of control operate in a closed-loop fashion, utilizing feedback and other information to make comparisons and modifications in the motor programs.

The programs represent a lower-order, open-loop method of control, initiated to carry out movements. Any activity that goes on for a reasonable period of time would probably activate both open-loop and closed-loop control from occasion to occasion. Stuart Klapp (1978) has reaffirmed Glencross' position, as he also recognizes the existence of hybrid systems of control in which both programmed and feedback control operate. After discussing mechanical and human systems, he concludes that "most systems at some level of analysis must be regarded as hybrid systems" (p. 231). The skilled performer, then, has developed adaptive strategies and component skills, enabling the potential shift to occur in a hybrid control system.

In contrast with skilled performers, novice performers have not received as much practice with a variety of movements, or perhaps even a particular movement. Therefore, their actions cannot be under programmed control. Rather, unskilled performers operate in a closed-loop fashion regardless of task demands, and their higher control centers are occupied with attending to the movement. As such, these performers cannot decide on the next movement in the sequence until the current one is completed. Thus, their performances tend to take an extended length of time, and this results in more errors occurring in the latter stages of movement sequences because the necessary response has not even been selected.

Control Over Response Selection and Execution

Difficulty in selecting and executing a response can lead to errors in response selection where the wrong response is chosen because the environment was misperceived. That is not to say that skilled performers do not commit errors in response selection, also. The difference is that the advanced performers are better prepared than the novice to choose the correct response owing to a greater experience with the task, more skills, and a greater capability to use appropriate strategies. However, regardless of experience, another type of performance error can occur, and at any skill level. These are errors in response execution, and they result from the musculature incorrectly enacting the movement commands. Once again, due to extended practice, highly-skilled individuals will tend to commit fewer of these errors than will their less-skilled counterparts.

The control of both types of error, selection and execution, involves the integrated functioning of processes associated with sensory storage, perception, the LTM, the STM, the movement generator, and feedback. Decisions for the selection of responses are made in the STM and are sequenced in the appropriate order in the movement generator. If an incorrect decision is made, or the programs are sequenced in anything but the proper order, then a performance error must occur. Similarly, if the programs are loaded correctly, but the movement generator incorrectly selects the musculature to perform the movement, then an error in execution will result. The difference in performance that is evidenced between high- and low-skilled individuals is related to the amount of their potential program control as well as the latency (time delay) within which either selection or execution errors can be corrected.

THE NATURE OF STRATEGIES AND INDIVIDUAL DIFFERENCES

It has been shown that strategies can be operative prior to involvement in an activity or the execution of a particular act, as in the case of preplanning or programming activities. Strategies can also be enacted during performance, assuming that the duration time of the act is long enough and adaptive behaviors are called for.

Generally speaking, strategies

(1) can be self-generated or imposed from an external source. Obviously, it is more desirable when they can be initiated appropriately under one's own direction.

(2) involve the development of rules or principles. They can be applied effectively to subsequent similar situations.

(3) require repeated attempts in situations, in resolving uncertainties and solving problems, if they are to become effective.

(4) are probably used differently by experts and beginners.

(5) are used effectively by experts; inefficiently by beginners.

(6) even differ among the highly skilled, owing to the nature of individual differences.

As Herbert Simon (1975) indicates, after showing that numerous distinct solution strategies are available in simple problem situations and different subjects learn different strategies,

> Different subjects may in fact learn different things in the same task environment, and a formal analysis of the environment can help define the range of possibilities. It can also help define differences in the demands that different methods of task performance place upon the subject (p. 268).

In other words, in any sporting situation, to extrapolate from Simon's work with the tower of Hanoi problem, a paper and pencil puzzle to solve, a number of strategies may be learned and alternatives may work equally well. A learning strategy or a teaching strategy must be matched according to a person's competences and cognitive style (preferred technique to approach and resolve a problem). It is probably rarely true that only one strategy can be applied to a learning of a particular task. It may be true that there is one best (optimal) strategy for a task.

A summary of the verbal learning research indicates that there can be large differences both among and within individuals in the strategies they select to cope with a particular task. People tend to think in different ways, even when the information presented is the same and the situational constraints are similar. "Skilled behavior is fixed in its objectives and yet flexible in its detail structure, in that the objectives may be achieved by a number of different strategies," writes D. Whitfield (1967, p. 157). Coaches and athletes need to analyze carefully the cognitive and psychological demands of an event or activity. The best strategies for achievement should be determined. At the same time, an analysis of the personal characteristics of the athlete might lead to some indication of situation-strategy compatibility or the lack of it.

PERFORMANCE AND LEARNING CONSIDERATIONS

When skills and tactics are acquired, in contrast to being performed in a contest, the "mental" approach may be quite different. It is true that practice conditions should simulate real conditions as much as possible for ideal preparation. But this assumes that the skills are indeed ready to be performed at a high level.

However, learning strategies and performance strategies may differ. In competitive performance, consciousness is tuned down, and activity flows. Deliberate conscious intervention switches on when appropriate, but if everything is going right, "things just seem to happen." This kind of comment occurs frequently from athletes on completion of an outstanding performance. Contest strategies are preplanned. Skills, tactics, and strategies have been learned well, so that deliberate attention to them may be unnecessary. Where this is not the case, special self-cueing devices may be appropriate. Also, when situations change, requiring alternative plans of action, conscious involvement fosters evaluative and adjustive activities.

During training sessions, the athlete attempts to perfect skills and tactics

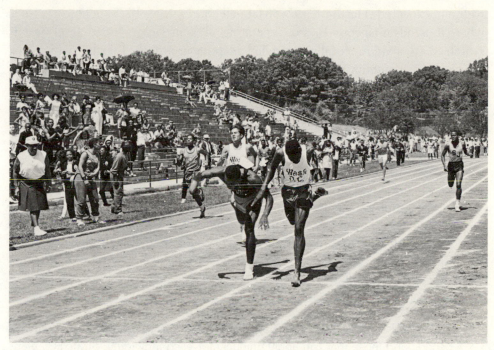

District of Columbia Recreation Department

Highly skilled performers demonstrate supreme physical conditioning, excellent movement mechanics, and the appearance of automatic behaviors.

as well as the use of primary and secondary strategies. A certain amount of trial and error is evidenced. More deliberate cognitive intervention occurs during training than in actual competitive events. Just as skills and techniques are mechanically and adaptively refined in practice, *thought and emotional processes need to trained as well.*

Gordon Pask (1975) suggests that both learning and performance strategies require the application of mental subroutines to achieve goals. But a learning strategy can help solve problems, such as deficiencies in the repertoire of performance strategies. A learning strategy is thus a plan for selecting performance strategies and then building or repairing them.

Performance demands suggest strategies that should be acquired. Some activities require more fixed responses; others more adaptive. Many athletes become "overtrained" in the performance of certain acts. That is to say, they may tend to respond too automatically. Usually associated with skill are higher levels of programming and organization, which give rise to rigidity in performance. When acts are highly practiced and well-learned, it is more difficult to respond to the unexpected (Hartnett, 1975; Mannell and Duthie, 1975). There are times when it is advantageous to stop operating at a preprogrammed level and to switch to an environmentally controlled adaptive approach. Flexibility in performance, which implies anticipation for the unexpected, needs to be practiced and perfected in training.

SUMMARY

Differences in skill level may be attributed to many factors, but in this chapter the emphasis was on the processing of information, learner strategies, and learning/performance. Stating it simply, higher-skilled performers process information more effectively and efficiently than the less skilled. They have learned pertinent strategies to enhance processing at different stages, from the inflow of information to the movement made in response to task demands. They have also learned how to direct their thoughts and emotional processes appropriately, prior to, during, and after an event.

The skilled can become more skillful when consideration is given to processes and strategies that can potentially govern learning and performance in general and those that can apply uniquely for each individual. Strategies, plans, and the formation of programs are closely allied to the production of skilled movement. Skilled behavior is evinced as a function of the sophistication of appropriate cognitions, a response repertoire, and the resources of the physical-emotional system.

REFERENCES AND SUGGESTED READINGS

Chi, M. T. H. Short-term memory limitations in children: capacity or processing deficits? *Memory and Cognition,* 1976, 4, 559–572.

Gallwey, W. T. *Inner tennis.* New York: Random House, 1976.

Gentile, A. M. and Nacson, J. Organizational processes in motor control. In Keogh, J. and Hutton, R. S. (eds.), *Exercise and sport reviews,* volume 4. Santa Barbara, Cal.: Journal of Publishing Affiliates, 1976.

Glencross, D. J. Control of skilled movements. *Psychological Bulletin,* 1977, 84, 14–29.

Hall, C. R. A review of encoding processes in verbal and motor memory. *Canadian Journal of Applied Sciences,* 1978, 3, 208–214.

Hartnett, O. M. Errors in responses to infrequent signals. *Ergonomics,* 1975, 18, 213–223.

Hearst, E. and Wierzbicki, M. Battle royal: psychology and the chessplayer. In Goldstein, J. H. (ed.), *Sports, games, and play: social and psychological viewpoints.* Hillsdale, N.J.: Erlbaum, 1979.

Housner, L. D. and Hoffman, S. J. *Imagery and short-term motor memory.* Paper presented at the annual meeting of the North American Society for the Psychology of Sport and Physical Activity, Tallahassee, Fla., May 1978.

Klapp, S. T. Reaction time analysis of programmed control. In Hutton, R. S. (ed.), *Exercise and sport sciences reviews,* volume 5. Santa Barbara, Cal.: Journal Publishing Affiliates, 1978.

Mannell, R. C. and Duthie, J. H. Habit lag: when "automatization" is disfunctional. *The Journal of Psychology,* 1975, 89, 73–80.

Newell, K. M. Some issues on action plans. In Stelmach, G. E. (ed.), *Information processing in motor control and learning.* New York: Academic Press, 1978.

Nideffer, R. M. *The inner athlete.* New York: Crowell, 1976.

Pask, G. *The cybernetics of human learning and performance.* London: Hutchinson, 1975.

Simon, H. A. On how to decide what to do. *The Bell Journal of Economics,* 1978, 9, 494–507.

Simon, H. A. The functional equivalence of problem solving skills. *Cognitive Psychology,* 1975, 7, 268–288.

Singer, R. N. *Motor learning and human performance: An application to motor skills and movement behaviors,* third edition. New York: Macmillan Publishing Co., Inc., 1980.

Singer, R. N. Motor skills and learning strategies. In O'Neil, H. F. (ed.), *Learning strategies.* New York: Academic Press, 1978.

Singer, R. N. and Gerson, R. F. Learning strategies, cognitive processes, and motor learning. In O'Neil, H. F. and Spielberger, C. D. (eds.), *Cognitive and affective strategies.* New York: Academic Press, 1979.

Spielberger, C. D., Gonzalez, H. P., and Fletcher, T. Test anxiety reduction, learning strategies, and academic performance. In O'Neil, H. F. and Spielberger, C. D. (eds.), *Cognitive and affective learning strategies.* New York: Academic Press, 1979.

Stuart, R. B. (ed.) *Behavioral self-management.* New York: Brunner/Mazel, 1977.

Underwood, G. (ed.) *Strategies of information processing.* New York: Academic Press, 1978.

Wenz, B. J. and Strong, D. J. An application of biofeedback and self-regulation procedures with superior athletes: the fine tuning effect. In Suinn, R. M. (ed.), *Psychology in sports: methods and applications.* Minneapolis, Minn.: Burgess, 1980.

Whitfield, D. Human skill as a determinate of allocation of function. *Ergonomics,* 1967, 10, 154–160.

Whiting, H. T. A. Overview of the skill learning process. *Research Quarterly,* 1972, 43, 266–294.

10

MOTOR LEARNING AND PROGRAMS OF PHYSICAL EDUCATION AND SPORT

At this stage in the book you should be quite familiar with the nature of learning skills, and should understand what situational and personal factors are of major influence. As a physical educator to be, or one already, you must be concerned with how students learn skills, and how they can learn them more expeditiously.

But physical education programs are guided under personal philosophies and situational constraints. Many potential outcomes can be attained by participants in physical education programs. The learning of skills is one outcome. Other outcomes are possible, too. In this chapter we will analyze possible goals of programs, and provide a perspective on the learning of skills in that context. Students (or athletes) are not merely assembly-line robots, to be trained mechanically and forgotten. They are to be nurtured, nourished, and guided in many ways.

The type of guidance offered by physical educators to students can be reckless or thoughtless, or structured from scientific underpinnings. Communication style is personal; it may even be artistic. Yet the content of physical education programs, what is taught, and the goals set and realized, should be associated with a concrete support base extracted from the scientific and philosophical evidence. In other words, there need not—should not—be a gap between a body of research information and the practical or real world in which it should be used. Bridging this potential gap will be discussed later on. First, let us turn to the possible goals of physical education programs.

GOALS OF PROGRAMS

Teachers cannot hope to achieve all possible goals in the limited time they spend with students. Priorities must be established. Once they are, certain goals can be emphasized over others with various activities, and students will have a better chance of having them realized. Generally speaking, teaching in physical education is oriented to influence one or a combination of the four following outcomes:

> **(1)** skill, knowledge, or fitness
> **(2)** socialization skills
> **(3)** personal factors
> **(4)** learning processes

Skill, knowledge, or fitness. In this approach, attention is focused on the efficient acquisition of specific skills, information, or fitness. Mastery and achievement are the major intentions with regard to student outcomes. Group and individualized instruction have been developed to guide students through learning material to intended attainment levels. Highly guided and prompted learning highlight this mode.

Socialization skills. Improved social relations, the ability to relate to others, is the theme of the approach. Experiences in human relations, communication, interaction, and understanding others underlie this approach in physical education.

Personal factors. The intention behind the personal focus is to use physical activity to develop personal qualities. Self-confidence, self-realization, self-concept, enjoyment, and satisfaction represent "personal states" that might be influenced. Likewise, responsibility for decisions and performance outcomes is taught to students. Students' intrinsic motivation toward activity selection and perseverance is another personalized attitude with which the teacher might be concerned.

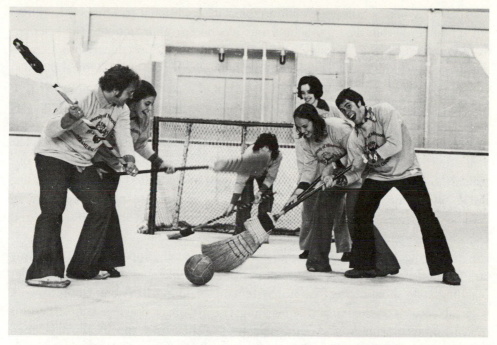

Featherkill Studios, Burnsville, MN

Learning skills and having fun can go together.

Learning processes. This approach focuses on student's learning abilities and processes. Techniques to help students analyze activities and situational demands, to use thought processes, to solve problems, and to create are stressed. Emphasis is on process rather than content, and individualized approaches and behaviors are encouraged.

The general teaching model used will influence instructional strategies and settings and, in turn, what goals are realized. One approach might emphasize the teacher's role and another the student's role as to decision-making and the nature of class activity. In any event, a teacher formulates (or should formulate) a priority order of objectives which, in turn, leads to a basic teaching model, while other models can be used on occasion to help fulfill lower-priority objectives.

A COMPARISON OF PROGRAMS

These teaching approaches to achieve intended outcomes suggest instructional alternatives. Each is suited to realizing certain objectives. Often styles are combined. All can and do produce learning. Some teachers look for alternatives in instruction, whereas others are comfortable with traditional techniques. In different schools or within the same school, one sees diverse approaches to the teaching of physical education. Although in recent years the trend in education in general has been toward individualized learning, the unwieldy size of the typical physical education class encourages teachers to assume a more dominant role in instructing for normative group behaviors while remaining sensitive to individual differences.

Some teachers attempt to reach broad-based educational and physical education objectives while others remain true to learning theory or behavioral principles. Still others operate on a loosely structured day-to-day basis. Many valid questions concerning student betterment have been raised by dedicated physical educators, but a satisfactory resolution still remains difficult because of discrepancies in general objectives, teaching techniques, interpretation and use of research and learning theory, and the process of putting it all together.

Regardless of the teaching method, it is usually apparent that the way any method is employed is very important. The implementation of a particular teaching style should reflect careful systematic planning. It is one thing to work with objectives or theory and something else to break down a course or unit into meaningful sequences. Are the objectives of the course specifically developed in behavioral terms? Can they be accurately evaluated to see if they are attained? Are they practical? Have limitations on space, equipment, time, and human resources been considered? If so, how? Are the students' beginning skills, characteristics, and attitudes specified and considered when formulating the program and its objectives?

Perhaps a major problem in the past was the attempt to determine one right way of teaching, as if such existed. A more realistic stance is to appraise a particular approach to teaching according to instructional goals and types of students involved.

VALUES IN THE LEARNING OF MOTOR SKILLS

Although we have dealt exclusively with the learning of motor skills in this book, many of the learning considerations addressed can be applied to the learning of anything: values, social skill, intellectual material, how to learn, and so on. Consequently, whatever your goals in teaching as a physical educator, it is expected that the material you have read on the preceding pages will be of some help in your efforts.

Learning of a meaningful nature must occur if a program is to have educational value, if it is to be recognized for its educational merits. Although a variety of learning outcomes can be taught for in a physical education program, as we have seen in the previous sections, perhaps at the heart of meaningful learning is the students' acquisition of a reasonable level of skill in a reasonable number of activities. Achievement in activities fosters further participation, promotes self-fulfillment, and can contribute to a higher self-concept. In other words, learning an activity can be either an end in itself or the means by which concomitant values may be derived—or both.

The attainment of a reasonable level of proficiency in an activity can serve many purposes for a student. It demonstrates an ability to gain competence in an endeavor. It shows a capability to meet challenges, and to overcome them. And if the experience is pleasurable and personally rewarding, the student will probably wish to participate more in the activity, in or out of school. Therefore, the learning of the motor skills associated with physical education curricula and athletic programs should be personally meaningful and enjoyable, efficiently realized, and productive as to goals attained.

UNDERSTANDING LEARNERS

Any educational program is beneficial to more participants when sensitivity is shown to individual differences. A humanistic approach is more humane: it respects individuals as individuals. Although a good portion of this book is dedicated to the proposition that there are generally applicable processes and behaviors that most people might use to advantage in a particular situation, an underlying warning was added that people differ quite a bit as well.

Consequently, we try to teach for the "average" learner in a group, using techniques and approaches compatible with what we know from the body of literature associated with the psychology of learning and teaching. And yet meaningful ways in which students differ need to be identified. Special instructional approaches must be considered. The goal in any program is for *all* students to achieve as close to their potential as possible. This means that the instructor's responsibilities are varied and extensive, for the burden of student learning lies on his/her shoulders.

There are times when the process of learning seems so simple; in fact, it should be simple. On other occasions, athletic activities appear almost impossible to master, even at a moderate level. Many personal, instructional, and situational factors contribute to a person's ease in acquiring skill in a particular activity. When such factors operate against a learner, they need to be remedied quickly.

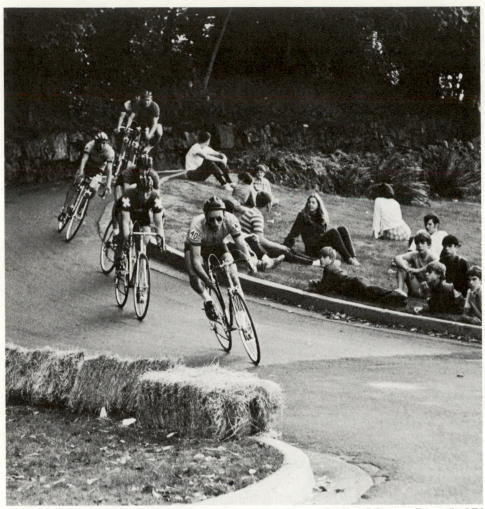

Featherkill Studios, Burnsville, MN

Physical skills allow people to test themselves and to derive a sense of satisfaction.

There are times when instruction should be kept plain, or in the acronym warning, KISS, of my old beloved Ohio State University friend, Spike Mooney:

Keep
It
Simple,
Stupid.

We must not over-teach and over-reach our students. We must not short-change them, either. More complex skills and directions have their place and time. Teachers who view teaching as an art and a science will probably demonstrate a more comprehensive understanding of what the learning process is all about. They will know what to do, and when to do it.

BRIDGING THE GAP: FROM RESEARCH TO PRACTICE

The expressing "bridging the gap" has become quite popular in education in recent years. There are teachers who believe that research is irrelevant and meaningless; that teaching is intuitive and personal. Therefore, to them, there is no gap to bridge. But even among those who agree that there should be a close relationship between the practice of teaching and a supportive scientific body of knowledge, many disagree as to who has the primary responsibility in "reaching out." Should the teacher-practitioner learn more about research and be able to translate it for personal use? Should the researcher-theorist write material more applicable for teaching situations? Whose responsibility is it to bridge the gap? Obviously, it would be nice if both parties reached out.

One purpose of teaching models, learning theories, and research is to suggest logical teaching styles that will best encourage and promote learning. There is no one accepted theory. Owing to the youthfulness of the psychology of learning, theories are incomplete, many questions are unresolved, a number of research findings are contradictory, and there is no particular behavioral technology to turn to. The suggestive evidence supports various popular teaching and learning strategies. However, there is no major solution or easy way out.

SUMMARY

The intention in this brief chapter has been to reflect about the philosophy of learning motor skills in the context of physical education programs. Philosophical issues were analyzed as to the intended outcomes of physical education curricula. Furthermore, the relationship of teaching and research was discussed. Teaching should be an art and science; it should be intuitive and personal, and yet reflect that what is known from research and theory.

REFERENCES AND SUGGESTED READINGS

Bain, L. Status of curriculum theory in physical education. *Journal of Physical Education and Recreation,* 1978, 49, 25–26.

Dunkin, M. J., and Biddle, B. J. *The study of teaching.* New York: Holt, Rinehart and Winston, 1974.

Joyce, B., and Weil, M. *Models of teaching,* second edition. Englewood Cliffs, N.J.: Prentice-Hall, 1980.

Locke, L. F. Research on teaching physical education: new hope for a dismal science. *Quest,* 1977, 28, 2–16.

Singer, R. N., and Dick, W. *Teaching physical education: a systems approach,* second edition. Boston: Houghton Mifflin Co., 1980.

11

AN OVERVIEW: LEARNING PRINCIPLES

It would be very convenient for the physical educator to be able to have a list of certain absolute truths or learning principles to follow. He or she could use these as handy guidelines in a particular teaching situation. Unfortunately, although we now know more about conditions that contribute to learning than ever before, it is difficult to construct many conclusive statements that would go unchallenged.

The reasons for this predicament are obvious. Learning is no simple matter. So many factors interact to influence the outcome of the learning situation that it is almost impossible to treat any aspect of the learning process without regard for all these factors. One of the greatest challenges in writing a book of this nature is to bring some sort of order to a description of the learning process out of so much ever-expanding research and theoretical evidence.

The attempt in this chapter will be to summarize learning principles, encompassing the many factors discussed in this book and elsewhere. The principles are based on an interpretation of the research evidence. It should be no means by assumed that they are founded on research findings that are in complete agreement. Also, no principles are final. These are meant as tentative operational guidelines, to be reinforced or modified by future research evidence.

For the sake of continuity, the principles set forth here are parallel to the major divisions of this book. Three categories of principles have been formed, which include General Learning Processes; Individual Differences; and Instructional Conditions.

_____ **POSSIBLE PROJECT** _____

Select any principle presented in this chapter, a topic of interest to you. Review research and textbooks and then arrive at some conclusion as to the principle stated here. Is the principle correctly stated? Do you believe it should be restated or modified?

The project format might include:

(1) An introduction to the problem (principle).
(2) A review of literature (any kind of learning matter, not necessarily only motor skills).
(3) Conclusions.
(4) Reference list.

The following are some suggested resources:

(1) *Research Quarterly*
(2) *Journal of Motor Behavior*
(3) *Perceptual and Motor Skills*
(4) *Psychological Abstracts*
(5) *Completed Research in Health, Physical Education, and Recreation*
(6) *Dissertation Abstracts*
(7) Other journals

Through the project you will gain experience in attempting to generalize from the research. You will also become more familiar with research approaches and findings in an area with which you have some concern. Finally, you may find that I misstated a principle—and everyone likes to find fault in another's work!

GENERAL LEARNING PROCESSES

1. *Learning* has been *defined* as a relatively permanent change in performance or behavioral potential resulting from practice or past experience in the situation. It is usually distinguished from developmental, transitory, and performance factors.

2. *Learning* and *performance* are not synonymous terms, for performance is a function both of an individual's past experience (learning) and other variables, mainly motivation. There are many occasions when, for various reasons, performance levels do not reflect the true amount of learning that has occurred. However, performance scores are the best indicators of learning as of the present time.

3. *Learning curves* are graphic representations of changes in behavior over time, as a result of practice under designated conditions.
   a. Great *irregularities* usually appear from person to person and from task to task when learning curves are examined. However, when averaged out over many people and possibly blocks of trials, any one of *four different types of curves* may be obtained: negatively accelerated, linear, S-shaped, or positively accelerated.
   b. Learning curves are *influenced* by: the treatment (experiences) given to people; performance artifacts and personal factors (fatigue, motivation, etc.); the type of task used (e.g., difficulty); the number of practice trials allowed; the type of measurement selected; and the number of scores used as the basis for each trial.

4. A *plateau*, which is a leveling off in performance after rapid improvement and which precedes another improvement stage, has rarely been obtained in experimental studies although empirical evidence points to the existence of this phenomenon.
   a. Possible *causes* of plateaus might be loss of interest, loss of novelty, loss of motivation; focus on wrong cues; fatigue, emotions; lack of physical readiness; low level of aspiration; lack of understanding of directions; and lack of ability to reorganize and adapt skills.
   b. During the difficult period of transition and task reorganization, patience and motivation must continue to prevail.

5. The *understanding of learning and performance* encompasses *three* major categories of factors: the learner, and consideration for individual differences; the learning process, and similarities among individuals; and situations, how practice and training conditions differentially influence the average learner and different types of learner(s).

6. A recurring issue is whether there is *one kind* of learning or *many*, and whether different categories of behavior need to be identified. The trend seems to be in the direction of considering the unique features of motor learning, along with those in common with other types of learning.

7. The *psychomotor domain* is *broad* and encompassing, and psychomotor behaviors are associated with many occupations, recretional endeavors, and daily routines.

8. Motor skills or tasks have been conveniently *categorized*, although without rigid and agreed-on criteria. Gross and fine tasks, continuous and discrete tasks, motion of person and object, self-paced, mixed-paced, and externally paced tasks, and open and closed skills have been described, with the possibility that alternative teaching/learning strategies may be applicable for different kinds of tasks.

9. *Skill* can be *described* in terms of speed, accuracy, form, efficiency, and adaptability, or any combination of these. It has been *defined* as the consistent degree of success in achieving an objective with efficiency and effectiveness. A *skill* consists of a specific set of responses to particular cues in certain situations, whereas *an ability* is a general trait that contributes to success in the performance of a number of skills.

10. *Skill* is a function of *input* (the reception and analysis of information), central processes (control and decisions), and *output* (motor functions).

11. It is fair to say that personal *structures and mechanisms* operate similarly across people, unless there is some type of impairment. *How* these structures and mechanisms are *used* differ among people, leading to learning and performance.

12. *Proficiency* is any complex activity *depends* on genetic factors, childhood experiences, the learning of specific skills and knowledge related to the activity, state of training, motivation, and guidance.

13. *Human control, behavioral, and processing systems* are likened in operation to a *computer*. Computers are designed to handle much information at one time and to produce an accurate output based on input and central decision-making processes. More elaborate operations can be demonstrated by more complexly designed computers. Similarly, more mature and experienced humans can produce performances superior to those produced by inexperienced ones.

    a. The human system is potentially *energized* upon the receipt of information (cues, stimuli) from *internal* (inside the person) or *external* (situational, environmental, task) factors by sense receptors. A certain amount of information will proceed through the system, to be processed and reacted to, while other information will be below the threshold value necessary for reaction.

    b. Upon the activation of the *senses*, information is detected or transmitted to the long-term memory store to make contact with previously stored, similar representations, to provide initial meaning to the preprocessed information.

    c. The *short-term memory* (STM) is the most significant mechanism in the system for operations performed on the information, and it is referred to as the *working* memory. It is there that information is rehearsed and organized and decisions are made about what to do with it. STM provides a temporary storage area for information, and decisions are made about immediate responses and/or the transfer of information into long-term memory (LTM) for future reference.

d. Information stimulates a *broad distribution in the brain* that is organized into a representational system. Changes do not occur in only one place in the brain.

e. *Programs of action* are selected, based on situational analysis and reference to pertinent information in the LTM. These programs, or plans, may be simple or complex, under nonvolitional or volitional control.

f. The *information-processing capabilities* of people are *limited*. There is just so much information that can be dealt with at one time. The use of *capacity* and the application of internalized *strategies* vary from individual to individual, resulting in performance differences.

g. The *arousal state* of the person as information is organized in his or her system will determine the effectiveness of the processing.

h. *Effector mechanisms* execute the movement and produce *response-produced feedback*, to be used during the movement to help regulate and control it, or afterward, in subsequent situations, depending on the speed and brevity of the movement. Feedback about performance outcomes also provides information that leads to expectations regarding future performance.

14. A person learns to become more *self-dependent*, instead of externally reliant, with the acquisition of skill. From signal detection to feedback, interpretations and decisions become more *self-generated*. This is to say, the novice requires assistance and looks to the guidance of the instructor for which cues to attend to and what response to make. With the acquisition of skill, the learner learns to interpret situations for himself or herself and to make appropriate decisions about behaviors.

15. Human systems operate *differentially* because of differences in abilities and capabilities, genetics, structure, emotional reactivity, developmental factors, previous instruction and experiences, motivations, environmental conditions, and sociocultural influences.

16. Developmental factors are important to consider in the learning process. One of these factors is the *optimal* period to acquire a skill. Successful skill attainment at maturity is not dependent on the earliness of instruction, but rather on its *timeliness*.

a. *Delay in experiences* or a *restriction* of them may have detrimental effects on learning later in life.

b. Although critical learning periods for certain behaviors have been experimentally verified with *animals*, we can only advance the theoretical premise that an optimal learning period exists for the learning of anything as far as *humans* are concerned. As to the acquisition of basic skills, i.e., crawling, walking, and so on, their sequence is fairly predictable although the specific age when each occurs varies from individual to individual.

c. It does appear as if many athletic skills can be introduced at an *earlier period* of life than once was thought possible.

17. From early childhood to maturity, human behavior becomes more *individualistic* rather than similar between organisms. The *interrelationships* of physical development factors and intellectual achievements are only slightly correlated with respect to school-aged children.

18. There is great difficulty in ascertaining the *optimal age* for skill in motor performances, for a person today demonstrates superior skills at earlier and later ages than ever before. Data on outstanding Olympic and professional athletes indicates the middle twenties as the general period in life when most male athletes reach their peaks in performance. Nevertheless, once maturational readiness is present for a given activity, diligent and correct training can lead to a high proficiency in that activity.

19. *Sex differences* in motor performance become more apparent with increasing age after early childhood. Boys typically accelerate in motor performance during the adolescent years while girls level off and even demonstrate performance decrements. These differences in performance can be explained by reasons other than merely anatomical and physiological dissimilarities between the sexes. With social approval and increased motivation, girls and women achieve much greater skill levels in a variety of sports.

20. *Genetic factors* limit potential performance, but there is quite a gap between the operational level of individuals and their theoretical limits.

a. Most human behavior is *learned*, rather than influenced by hereditary factors. Therefore, the physical educator can influence behavior by providing students with directed desirable environmental experiences. Genetically imposed limitations can be *overcome* to a reasonable extent through individual learning programs and sensitive instruction.

b. Environmental experiences actually determine the level of skill attainment; thus, motor skill is dependent on the *interaction* of both genetics and environment.

21. *Young children* are at a *disadvantage* in learning certain skills, as compared to more mature individuals, but a consideration of certain factors can lead to more fruitful learning outcomes with motor skills.

a. A child is *limited* in *information-processing capabilities. Distraction* occurs easily and attention span is poor. *Gross movements* precede fine movements.

b. Children's *learning* can be *improved* if learning activities involve more *gross muscle movements, simplified actions,* and *minimal cues* to which to respond. Verbal cues by an outsider should be simple and limited. One or two of the cues most relevant to the child's developmental level should be emphasized. Too many cues are confusing to a child.

c. Learning activities should be *modified* to accommodate the stage of a child's *development,* or the child should be provided with special instruction that might aid the processing of information—from perception and selective attention to STM, to decision-making, to response integration, to feedback.

d. The child's need to achieve is apparent, and *failure* results in frustration, loss of motivation, and little desire to continue the experience.

e. Learning experiences should be *enjoyable* and *successful.* With success, increasing difficulty of the activity is appropriate; with failure, reverting to more simplified activity is a necessity.

22. A child learning a new activity can be considered on occasion to possess many of the *same problems* as the beginning adult learner, and yet there are differences; these are primarily associated with the cumulative learning effect, which favors the adult. Children appear to develop an information-processing *capacity* similar to that of adults, but the *effective use* of this capacity must be learned, to free it in terms of selective attention, anticipation, and decision-making and response-execution possibilities.

INDIVIDUAL DIFFERENCES

1. There are too many *personal* (or *individual difference*) factors to describe here that can potentially influence learning and performance levels. Many of these personal factors influence all forms of learning, and some are more particularly associated with psychomotor behaviors. Body build, physical measures (strength, endurance, speed, etc.), motor abilities, previously learned skills, and fear of danger in performance are factors associated with psychomotor behaviors.

2. *Characteristics* and *aptitudes* (the learner status prior to a learning experience) and specific *instructional conditions interact* to produce the most beneficial

outcomes. The optimum learning condition varies from person to person and must be determined on an individual basis.

3. *Normative data* are often calculated with regard to abilities, aptitudes, and learning level, but *individual scores vary* around the mean score; the extent of that variation is determined by the nature of the sample, the test, and the testing situation.

4. Individuals progress in skill acquisition at varying rates of speed, but *early success* does not indicate *later achievement*. Some students are slow learners and others are fast learners of a particular task, which requires the teacher to allow each individual the amount of time it takes for the learning of each task.

   a. *Extended practice* is of more value to those learners who demonstrate initial difficulty with the task. The relationship between initial and final status, although somewhat predictable for simple tasks, is not nearly as correlated in the case of complex tasks.

   b. With practice there is an apparent change in the *pattern* of abilities contributory to achievement. The *abilities* important for early success in a given motor task are not necessarily the same as those contributing to later proficiency. The teacher might emphasize the cues consistent with the specific abilities contributing most to success during each of the various stages of skill acquisition.

5. *Tests* that presumably assess motor ability, motor educability, and motor capacity have *limited value* for their stated purposes. Rather than thinking in terms of the existence of a general motor ability within a person, it is more useful to expect that each person possesses different levels of a number of abilities based on genetic and experiential factors.

6. Much laboratory research, artifically contrived, has tended to support the idea of *task specificity* rather than *task generality*. *Prediction* of task performance from performance on another task is usually inadequate, and achievement in activities is somewhat specific to the person and the activity. There are exceptions, of course. Success in real-life endeavors is dependent on existing abilities and capabilities brought to the learning situation, but no matter how great the original ability, *task-specific practice* is required for highly skilled behaviors.

7. *Success* in many sport skills is determined by:

   a. experience and intensive practice in a wide range of motor skills, especially in childhood;

   b. genetic factors, continuous motivation; and

   c. the relatedness of the skills to be learned to each other.

8. *Psychomotor abilities* have been deduced from logical reasoning or factor-

analytic studies, but an *acceptable taxonomy* or description has yet to be developed.

9. *Abilities* and *tasks* related to coordination, kinesthesis, balance, and speed of movement (reaction time, movement time, response time) have been of the greatest concern to motor learning researchers. Tests that primarily measure each of these factors have *not correlated well* with each other; i.e., test scores on coordination tasks seem to be somewhat independent of each other. It is probably impossible to tap only one ability in one test. However, many of these tasks have provided important information in regard to the learning processes and have aided in the ultimate prediction of activity performance in certain cases.

10. *Reaction time* and *movement time* are related but dissimiliar neuromuscular functions, and the correlations between them are not high. In other words, success in these acts, which work in various combinations in many motor skills, depends on different factors.

   a. Athletes in certain sports as well as people who practice reacting quickly usually have *faster* reaction times and movement times than nonathletes.

   b. A person can react more quickly to *touch* or *sound stimuli* than to *visual stimuli*. If a faster reaction is desired, it would be best to consider the nature of the stimuli and to choose stimuli that will facilitate the process.

   c. Reaction times become longer if *fatigue* has set in; if the person is reacting to *complex stimuli*, or if the individual is older or younger than the *second decade* of life (the twenties). Performance in tasks dependent to a great extent on reactions declines when any one or a combination of these circumstances is present.

11. There is no general *kinesthetic sense*. It is *specific* to the test and the part of the body involved in the skill. Kinesthesis is apparently related to successful motor performance, and like balance, coordination, and other abilities, must be developed specifically for a particular task.

12. Although *balancing ability* is important for athletic success, the performances of individuals in different tests of static and dynamic balance do not correlate highly. Specific sports probably require *specialized balancing abilities*. Therefore, this ability must be developed specifically for each activity.

13. *Coordination* is required for many skills, ranging from positioning and precision laboratory tasks to the performance of athletic activities. Coordination should not be thought of as a unitary factor, allowing individuals to achieve successfully across a wide assortment of tasks. This ability, like balance, must be developed *specifically* for the task at hand.

14. *Form* in performance is an individual matter. Good form, based on the latest mechanical, anatomical, and kinesiological evidence, is to be strived

for in the beginning. Individual differences, especially in body structures and proportions, necessitate allowing for many styles of skill execution. Therefore, learners should not be cast in a mold but rather allowed to express themselves within the limitations of their structures.

15. *Personal limitations,* such as sensory handicaps, perceptual handicaps, cognitive handicaps, and learning disorders should be recognized as possible sources of learning and performance problems. Special accommodating instructional procedures may need to be implemented.

16. Motor learning and performance are handicapped if *physical qualities,* such as strength, speed, and endurance necessary for the skilled movement are not well-developed. It is important that these qualities, especially as they relate to the task at hand, be developed to a reasonable degree.

17. *Emotional states* accompany motor learning and performance; some of them are inhibitive and others facilitative.

   a. People with *high anxiety* levels generally perform worse than those low in anxiety on *complex motor tasks,* such as required in the more advanced stages of most sports.

   b. *Stressful situations* are more disruptive to the learning of *complex tasks* than simple tasks. Evidently, then, greater sensitivity to the students on the part of the teacher is needed during the learning of more difficult motor skills.

18. The *level of expectation* or *level of aspiration* we set for ourselves in a given situation determines our success or failure and is a result of past successes and failures in the situation.

   a. *High, specific,* but *attainable goals* of intended achievement result in higher levels of performance.

   b. *Success* results in a rise of the aspiration level; *failure,* in a lowering of this level.

   c. *Success* is more *influential* than failure on the aspiration level. The learner should experience a reasonable amount of success if his or her motivation is to remain high and continue to rise.

19. The types of attributions we make (the reasons we give to ourselves as to what influenced our performance) are related to our level of achievement and persistence.

   a. A high *achievement motivated individual* is one who generally *attributes* success to high ability and high effort, failure to low effort.

   b. A *person low in achievement motivation* generally attributes success to good luck or task ease and failure to low ability.

   c. Persistent individuals attribute failure to lack of effort, an unstable and therefore changeable factor.

    d. Non-persistent individuals tend to quit when failing because they attribute failure to a lack of ability, which is a stable and non-changeable factor.

20. The learner is *totally* involved in any learning experience, and skill attainment might very well be related to such personal factors as physical characteristics, motor abilities, acuity of the senses, perceptual abilities, cognitions, and emotional status. All these variables must be considered for every individual and for every task.

21. A person's *behavior* in a given situation is more *complex* than simply the result of conditioning processes in operation. Responses are affected by many sociopsychological factors; namely, a person's attitudes, values, and personality in general, as well as the family, friends, and society.

INSTRUCTIONAL CONDITIONS

1. There is *no single method of instruction* appropriate for all teachers, for all students, and for all skills, although there are certain general techniques that seem to be beneficial for most students.

2. *Learning environments* can be *modified* in many ways if consideration is shown for learning-outcome objectives, the nature of the activities, and the characteristics of the learners. Physical environments can be varied, cues and feedback manipulated, and training procedures altered. Practice conditions can be consistent with what appear to be "accepted learning principles."

3. *Practice* alone does not lead to perfect performance. Errors may be practiced and perpetuated, or boredom may set in from mere repetition. Practice is beneficial if a number of factors are operating.
   a. *Attention* to relevant cues improves performance, and the learner should be directed with those cues whenever possible.
   b. *Intent to improve* leads to better performance.
   c. Rather than artificial practice activities, such as slowing down the responses demanded for the sake of concentrating on accuracy, practice should approximate ultimately desired movements as nearly as possible. Practice sessions should *simulate* test or contest situations.
   d. Practice should be of sufficient *quality* and *duration* to ensure the development of skill.

4. A number of considerations can be identified with regard to the learner's *state of preparedness to learn*. Obviously, the more the learner is predisposed to learn, the greater the presence of an ideal receptive state, and the probability of favorable learning outcomes is increased.

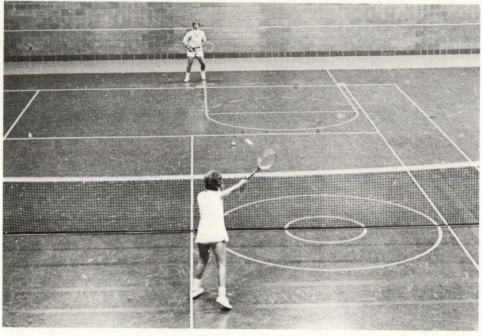

Featherkill Studios, Burnsville, MN

Quality practice leads to better performance.

5. *Meaningful goals* and intentions are important prerequisites, as are purposes. The meaningfulness of the task, especially as perceived by the learner, serves as a source of motivation.
   a. *Developmental readiness*, the possession of ideal personal qualities to tackle impending responsibilities, must be present to match task demands.
   b. *Psychological readiness* implies the presence of an appropriate psychological set and motivation to learn. Emotions must be matched to task demands, as an ideal emotional level enhances learning and performance.
6. There are many ways to *communicate the idea* of the nature of the material or the skill to be learned.
   a. Various approaches are available: verbal and written directions, visual forms (live models or filmed demonstrations), and, on occasion, the manipulation of passive limbs and body.
   b. On occasion learning rules or strategies, or principles of performance, are taught, with the hope that they will lead to greater insight, understanding, and learning of the content to be introduced.
   c. The communication of an act intended to be learned is effective when it stimulates the formation of an internalized image of the act to be

produced. Obviously, the quality of the instructional approach and the receptivity of the student will have a great deal to do with understanding and performance.

7. The *capacity* to process information at any stage depends, to a great extent, on *attentional processes*. Attention is related to such states as arousal and concentration, although distinctions can be made.

    a. The dominant concept of attention for many years was the *single-channel model*, although in more recent years, multichannel and other types of models have been proposed to describe human information-processing (attentional) capabilities.

    b. On the basis of studies dealing with divided attention (dual task or secondary task loading paradigms), it would appear that a number of human possibilities exist, depending on the attentional demands of simultaneously presented tasks.

8. The introduction of learning *cues* and *aids* can facilitate the acquisition of skill. They serve to *simplify* learning situations and task demands, to help *communicate* what is to be learned.

    a. The ability to learn and perform motor skills may very well be related to being able to *apply external* (instructor-provided) *words* and *internal words* (verbal mediation) to these acts. In order to perform effectively the learner must be able to *associate* certain *movement patterns* with *verbal cues*.

    b. Although it is logical to assume that an understanding of *mechanical principles* as applied to motor acts should benefit the performer, this premise does not always hold true. The best that can be said at this time is that some individuals prosper more, some less, when their time is devoted learning mechanical principles. It must be remembered that time spent learning mechanical principles takes away from time spent in participation. The learning of principles may transfer to the learning of motor acts, but not necessarily.

    c. Cues relevant to the learner's *stage of proficiency* should be emphasized. *Visual cues*, especially in the initial stages of learning, appear to be very important sense cues in the acquisition of many motor skills. *Kinesthetic cues* are important at higher levels of skill proficiency.

    d. *Visual cues*, whether of the natural type or teacher-constructed, have usually been of great service to individuals learning motor skills. *Specific*, *precise*, and *nearby* visual cues are easier to attend to than general, vague, and more removed cues.

    e. Many *training devices* have been developed to supplement teacher instruction. Research, although sparse, on the various types of training equipment indicates the value of some of these over and beyond the usual teaching procedures. Ball machines, simulated golf courses, and the like provide the learner with the means of learning and maintaining skill. They also may help to eliminate errors and hasten the learning process.

f. *Visual aids*, in such forms as motion pictures, slides, and force–time graphs, are somewhat valuable, but research does not indicate their conclusive worth as teaching aids. However, they probably provide supplementary information, enliven teacher routines, and motivate students.

g. Although *music* has served as a stimulator, motivator, or relaxer of behavior in some other areas, the influence of musical sounds and tempi on motor performance has yet to be scientifically verified.

h. Any *artificial* condition, such as special cues, aids, or simulators, should be *eliminated* from practice routines as soon as possible. Otherwise learners may become too dependent on them.

9. The performers' disparate *level of skill* will require varied learning considerations on the part of the instructor.

a. Especially with the beginner, his or her *attention* should be directed to understanding *purposes* and *goals* associated with the activity.

b. *Physical activity* should be emphasized and maximized in the early stages of motor learning. This is especially true with younger children and complex skills.

c. For most beginners, *shorter practice periods* spaced more often are preferable to fewer but more extended practice sessions.

d. New skills should be taught in such a way that the learner *performs in practice* the way he or she is expected to in the actual situation.

e. *Critical details* of performance should be analyzed with the advanced learner rather with than the beginner.

f. Advanced learners benefit more than beginners from extensive and intensive *verbal instructions*.

g. Advanced learners, because of their greater skill development and higher motivation levels, can *concentrate* for longer periods of time in practice than beginners.

10. *Motivation* is related to and influences achievement, persistence in practice, task selection, and effort. Motivation is also a factor in explaining variable performances.

a. Higher motivation impedes progress in complex tasks. The best performance is attained by individuals with intermediate motivation or arousal, as described in the inverted U hypothesis. Evidently, there is an optimal motivation level for each task, and for each person.

b. *Better-learned skills* are less prone to be disrupted by manipulated environmental conditions; i.e., different motivational conditions are more influential during the initial and unstable stages of learning.

c. Motivation may stem from intrinsic or extrinsic sources. *Intrinsic* refers to doing something for its own sake, and *extrinsic*, to material gains. Both types of motivation can improve performance, but intrinsic motivation is preferable and supposedly a more effective, sustaining type of motivation.

d. *Intrinsic* sources of motivation are thought to be more desirable than extrinsic sources of motivation. On occasion, rewards may *undermine* intrinsic motivation, especially when the latter is already present to a sufficient degree.

e. Varying the amount of *reward* appears to result in a change of performance in favor of the reward with the greatest magnitude.

f. *Reinforcement* increases the probability that the desired act will occur. The use of reinforcers as a powerful means of shaping behavior has been recognized for many years, with consideration for the type, schedule, and frequency of reinforcers. Their use is especially favored with those learners who do not seem to have much of an interest in learning a motor activity. Random reinforcement is a more effective continuing form of motivation than constant reinforcement.

g. Different people may respond differentially to motivational techniques, thus the *appropriate* type must be applied to each one's learning situation at the right time if the most favorable results are to be observed.

h. Motivation does not automatically increase with *success* and decrease with *failure*, for much depends on the difficulty of the task and the anxiety level of the performer. There are many instances when failure, instead of discouraging the learner, heightens his or her motivation.

i. When learning a new task, learners should experience as much *success* as possible in the early stages, before failure.

j. *Reward* is a more stable and stronger influence for desired behavior than *punishment*. The learner is more apt to perform more effectively when rewarded or acknowledged positively for correct responses.

11. *Four dimensions* of motor activities may be considered in regard to motivation: complexity, physical demands, appeal, and meaningfulness. More complex activities require less arousal level than simpler ones for their execution, except when simple tasks are to be repeated over and over again. More arousal is needed for the execution of "physical tasks," those in which the mechanics of movement are relatively simple or else well learned, and power,

speed, strength, or endurance are the primary bases for success. When activities are appealing, interesting, and meaningful to learners, motivation will be present to a more desirable degree than when they are absent.

12. Individuals vary in many dimensions, with implications for *motivational* considerations. To be considered are: under- or overachievement; level of aspiration or expectations in performance; need to achieve; need for social approval; need to avoid failure or to avoid success; level of anxiety; future orientation, or personal goals; internal or external locus of control; extrinsic and intrinsic motivation; and self-concept.

13. Various *conceptual approaches* to the study of motivation have resulted in different research paradigms, emphases, and conclusions. *Behavioristic* approaches tend to emphasize reinforcements and situational control over the learner. *Humanistic* approaches are oriented to inner-directed and self-determined behavior: helping people to help themselves. Approaches in *cognitive psychology* emphasize personal expectations in performance and interpretations (attributions) of performance outcomes.

14. *Achievement motivation programs* are related to the cognitive psychology school of thought, as intrinsic motivation for an activity is encouraged. An attempt is made to reach the attitudes and thoughts of learners, to develop a sense of responsibility in learners.

15. A number of *situational considerations* lead to *programs* or *activities* an instructor could initiate to influence motivation: the use of rewards and reinforcers; punishment; the use of knowledge of results of performance; the establishment of learner goals and expectations; the development and use of instructor objectives; competition; cooperation; instructor enthusiasm; effective leadership style and communication; interesting and meaningful training procedures; student involvement in goal setting, program development, and decision making; the development of learners' intrinsic strategies; learner feelings of control over self and over task outcomes; the learner's development of self-image, confidence, and self-worth; the application of knowledge of results of performance outcomes; successful learner experiences; and increased student responsibilities in the learning program.

16. People make *attributions* (perceived causes) for their performance outcomes; these, in turn, can influence their expectations for achievement when confronted with the same situation in the future. It is more desirable to attribute your performance to *internal causations* (energy expended and ability level) than to external causations (task difficulty and luck). Experiences should be established that lead to more successes, more objective attributions, and, in turn, better performances.

17. The *administration of practice sessions* affects the learning and, more probably, the performance of skills.
    a. It appears that *shorter practice* periods with *shorter rest* periods extended over a longer period of time are most effective for the acquisition of a number of motor skills.
    b. As to the learning of a skill in one given practice period, *distributed practice* exerts a more positive influence on performance than *massed practice*. This is evident because although immediate skill acquisition is favored under distributed practice, tests of later retention demonstrate little difference in performance between initially massed and distributed practice groups.
18. As to *whole versus part* methods of instruction, simple skills should be taught by the whole method whereas complex skills require some sort of breakdown.
    a. Task *complexity* and *organization* should be considered. With a *low degree of difficulty* and *high task organization* (interrelatedness of component tasks), the whole method appears to be preferable to the part method for skill acquisition.
    b. *More intelligent* people are likely to fare better under the whole method of instruction.
19. Motor skills can be learned to some degree without the benefit of *overt physical practice*.
    a. *Mental* or *image* practice, which is task rehearsal in the mind, yields better performance in a motor skill than no practice at all.
    b. *Physical practice* is more effective than mental practice, and the combination of mental-physical practice is slightly inferior or equal to physical practice alone. Although active participation is necessary to promote learning, evidently a certain amount of practice time can be spent in mental rehearsal without a loss of proficiency.
20. Although *drill* is satisfactorily used as a means for strengthening certain acts, a *problem-solving approach* may have much potential for the learning situation, especially in reaching objectives unattainable under the drill method. Particular learning situations warrant either one or the other. As an example, drill is effective for self-paced skills performed in stable environments. Greater flexibility in thought and movement, or problem solving, is associated with open-paced skills performed in changing, unpredictable environments.
21. *Knowledge of results* (KR) or *external feedback,* is extremely important in the learning process, especially in the *early* stages. There is usually some internal feedback available to the performer of motor skills. When feedback

is not available to or not used properly by the learner, KR should be supplied.

    a. Supplementary feedback may be *provided* during or immediately after performance, after performance at some designated time, and in various forms. It may serve not only as information to guide the learner, but as a source of *motivation* or *reinforcement* as well.

    b. Higher levels of performance are reached when KR is *specific* and *immediate.*

22. Learning is built upon previous learnings; hence, transfer potential exists from them for most of the things we attempt to learn. *Transfer,* which is the influence of a learned task on one to be learned, underlies almost all of learning. It is rare, if ever, that one learns something completely new.

    New tasks require a different patterning of the movements usually already found in the performer's repertoire of learned movements.

    a. Behavior and performance are influenced by *previous experiences;* in a given situation, positive, negative, or zero transfer may occur from prior to present learnings. The present learning situation and the student's past learning experiences should be analyzed in order to understand better how he or she will perform.

    b. If transfer is to occur successfully, the *desirability* of the transfer must be taught. Transfer will more probably occur when *relationships, resemblances,* and *concepts* between two learning situations are explained and demonstrated for the learner.

    c. Greater *resemblance* between task elements, between their respective stimuli and responses, results in a greater amount of *positive transfer.* When the new learning situation contains *stimuli similar* to the old situation but requires a *new response, negative transfer* occurs.

    d. Transfer is influenced by such factors as *amount of practice* on a prior related task, *method of training,* and *intent* of transfer.

    e. *Learning how to learn,* which involves learning the technique of attacking a particular kind of problem, is another aspect of transfer that leads to improvement to a greater degree than merely learning content.

    f. The effect of *initial-learned-task difficulty* on other tasks to be learned is uncertain. When the learning is concerned only with the nature of the response, the degree of transfer from a difficult task to an easy task is greater than from an easy task to a difficult one. Possibly, learning should progress from the simpler to the more complex conditions if an appropriate response is required to a continually changing and unpredictable pattern of stimuli.

23. A transfer of previously learned related skills and information will be more likely to occur when *relationships* between the past and present are under-

stood by the learner. Every effort should be made to communicate similarities to facilitate present learning.

    a. Learners should be prepared to practice in the context that more likely *resembles* testing conditions.

    b. A *warm-up* to refamiliarize learners with the situation is necessary after lay-offs. It helps to reorient the learner to the situational demands and the necessary responses.

24. *Gross motor skills* are usually *retained* for a longer time span than any other types of learning materials. Such skills are typically somewhat unique, they are overlearned, and retention is interferred with to a minimal extent.

    a. Material should be well-organized for the benefit of the learner, so there will be ease in internally organizing it for storage and retrieval purposes.

    b. More *meaningful* material is retained better by the learner. Therefore, the teacher should ensure that each newly introduced task is understood and has meaning to the student. Meaningful practice on meaningful tasks increases retention probability.

    c. *Overlearning* of a skill results in more effective retention.

    d. The learning and retaining of a particular response may very well be affected by what is learned either before or after training on this response, especially when it is of a related nature. *Proactive inhibition and retroactive inhibition* refer to the negative effects of these situations. Information on the student's activities prior to the learning of a given skill and afterwards might provide keener insight into performance expectancies for this student on this skill.

    e. Forgetting probably is due not merely to the *passage of time*, but rather to the *intervening* events between practice and recall. With fewer intervening events, retention should be better.

    f. With most *serially-learned* material, that which is learned first is retained best, the last learned is mastered second best, whereas the middle is last to be retained.

    g. *Continuous* tasks have been found to be retained more effectively than discrete tasks.

25. *Reminiscence*, a performance increase after a rest interval, has been obtained in many studies investigating the occurrence of this phenomenon. It appears as if massed practice tends to lead to greater reminiscence effects.

THE APPLICATION OF LEARNING PRINCIPLES

The compilation of this list of learning principles, or perhaps any inventory, in incomplete and subject to criticism. A statement is difficult to make without qualification. However, the preceding list of generalizations, although subject to change and certainly not definitive or completely true, represents an attempt to present in outline form the large body of knowledge relevant to learning; more specifically, the learning of motor skills.

The list of learning principles, if it may be called that, casts aside the camouflage and psychological jargon in an attempt to present isolated and in many instances unrelated statements. It is meant to serve as a guideline for the physical educator and not to be quoted out of context. It would be best in many cases to explore the principle of interest at greater depth before applying it to a given situation. The list itself represents the gleaning of information from countless journals and books. These publications are coming off the presses at such a tremendous rate that it is almost impossible to keep up with the latest findings and views in related learning areas.

Learning principles, constructed from the research evidence, should serve as the framework for any learning theory. The value and validity of any theory lies in its ability to incorporate all these more or less accepted statements and to apply them to explaining and predicting human behavior.

Physical educators are responsible for understanding and applying learning principles if they are to be effective teachers. They benefit from the efforts of researchers and theorists. Their goal should be to apply those learning principles that have the greatest probability of being successful in the situations they face. The mere consideration of all the possible factors that might interact to affect the performance of a group implies a great understanding of and sensitivity to the learning process. After considering individual differences as well, teaching will be even more effective.

Perhaps one of the greatest difficulties in teaching consistently with learning principles is the impracticality of distinguishing individuals from a group. Although certain principles generally apply to groups at large, individuals do learn at different speeds with different incentives, attitudes, and interests, and with varying degrees of developed abilities. Much depends on the desired objective: meeting group standards or individual achievement and satisfaction.

Another concern is the application of principles mainly derived from controlled laboratory experiments in which isolated novel tasks and a limited number of random and representative subjects are used. Sometimes experimental evidence conflicts with commonly accepted practices. How many of us wish to teach in a manner that contradicts our own common sense? Unfortunately, it is this situation precisely that hampers progress, for the instructor will never know if something works until he or she attempts to put it into practice.

Teaching and learning efficiency accompanies practice of a kind and under conditions consistent with scientific evidence. It is hoped that the list of learning principles, as well as the contents of this book, will be of value to the physical educator, the coach, or anyone else interested in and dedicated to improving human learning and performance in motor skills.

AUTHOR INDEX

SUBJECT INDEX

A

Abilities, 58
    cognitive and motor, 93
    generality vs. specificity issues, 92–93,
       171–172
    and learning, 88–89
    motor, 92
    and skills, 58
Accuracy and speed tradeoff, 124–126
Anticipation, 139
Arousal, 96, 144–145
Attention, 138–144, 197–199
Attributions, 160

B

Balance, 63–65
Behaviorism, 23–24

C

Children, 96–100
Cognitive processes, 188–190
Cognitive psychology, 25
Concentration, 139–140, 140–141
Control processes, 189, 200–203
    central, 200–303
    external, 90
    peripheral, 200–203
    self, 90
Coordination, 65, 67
Cybernetics, 27

D

Design of experiments, 49–52
Developmental considerations, 96–100, 148–149
Distribution of practice, 128–129

E

Emotions (*see* Arousal)
Error measurement, 37
    absolute error, 37
    constant error, 37
    variable error, 37
Experimental approach, 39–42

F

Feedback, 75–76, 148, 165–168, 199–200
Form, 94–95

G

General motor ability, 92–93
    all-round athletes, 93
    concepts, 92–93
    specificity issues, 92–93
    tests of, 92
Gestaltism, 25
Goal-setting, 116–118
Guided learning, 126–128

H

Hierarchical control systems, 29–30

I

Image formation, 116
Imagery, 116, 122
Individual differences, 94, 203–206
Information processing, 26–27, 135–136, 193–194
Instruction, 103
Instructional design, 104–108

242